Plastic Surgery Emergencies
Principles and Techniques

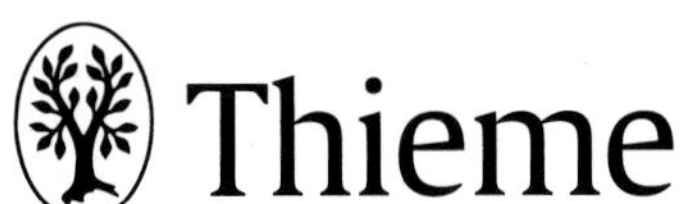

Plastic Surgery Emergencies
Principles and Techniques

Jamal M. Bullocks, MD
Assistant Professor
Division of Plastic Surgery
Michael E. Debakey Department of Surgery
Baylor College of Medicine
Texas Medical Center
Houston, Texas

Patrick W. Hsu, MD
Chief Resident
Division of Plastic Surgery
University of Medicine and Dentistry of New Jersey
Robert Wood Johnson Medical School
Camden, New Jersey

Shayan A. Izaddoost, MD, PhD
Division of Plastic Surgery
Michael E. Debakey Department of Surgery
Baylor College of Medicine
Texas Medical Center
Houston, Texas

Larry H. Hollier Jr., MD, FACS
Associate Professor
Division of Plastic Surgery
Michael E. Debakey Department of Surgery
Baylor College of Medicine
Texas Medical Center
Houston, Texas

Samuel Stal, MD, FACS
Professor and Chief
Division of Plastic Surgery
Michael E. Debakey Department of Surgery
Baylor College of Medicine
Texas Medical Center
Houston, Texas

Thieme
New York • Stuttgart

Thieme Medical Publishers, Inc.
333 Seventh Ave.
New York, NY 10001

Vice President, Production and Electronic Publishing: Anne T. Vinnicombe
Managing Editor: Owen Zurhellen IV
Vice President, International Marketing and Sales: Cornelia Schulze
Chief Financial Officer: Peter van Woerden
President: Brian D. Scanlan
Production Editor: Print Matters
Illustrator: Mike de la Flor
Cover Illustrator: Cara Ryan Downey, MD
Compositor: Thomson Digital
Printer: Everbest Printing Company

Library of Congress Cataloging-in-Publication Data

Plastic surgery emergencies : Jamal M. Bullocks ... [et al.].
p. ; cm.
Includes index.
ISBN 978-1-58890-670-0 (Americas : alk. paper) –
ISBN 978-3-13-145241-2 (Rest of world : alk. paper)
1. Surgery, Plastic. 2. Surgical emergencies. I. Bullocks, Jamal M.
[DNLM: 1. Reconstructive Surgical Procedures—methods. 2. Emergency Treatment—methods. 3. Wounds and Injuries—surgery. WO 600 P7114 2008]
RD118.P5363 2008
617.9'52—dc22

2007044537

Important note: Medical knowledge is ever-changing. As new research and clinical experience broaden our knowledge, changes in treatment and drug therapy may be required. The authors and editors of the material herein have consulted sources believed to be reliable in their efforts to provide information that is complete and in accord with the standards accepted at the time of publication. However, in view of the possibility of human error by the authors, editors, or publisher of the work herein or changes in medical knowledge, neither the authors, editors, or publisher, nor any other party who has been involved in the preparation of this work, warrants that the information contained herein is in every respect accurate or complete, and they are not responsible for any errors or omissions or for the results obtained from use of such information. Readers are encouraged to confirm the information contained herein with other sources. For example, readers are advised to check the product information sheet included in the package of each drug they plan to administer to be certain that the information contained in this publication is accurate and that changes have not been made in the recommended dose or in the contraindications for administration. This recommendation is of particular importance in connection with new or infrequently used drugs.

Some of the product names, patents, and registered designs referred to in this book are in fact registered trademarks or proprietary names even though specific reference to this fact is not always made in the text. Therefore, the appearance of a name without designation as proprietary is not to be construed as a representation by the publisher that it is in the public domain.

Printed in China
5 4 3 2 1

ISBN 978-1-58890-670-0

Contents

Foreword

"The man who graduates today and stops learning tomorrow is uneducated the day after."

—*Newton D. Baker Jr.*

When I was asked to write a foreword for this book *Plastic Surgery Emergencies*, I must confess, my first thought was "Is another book truly necessary?" But after reading it, I am both honored and flattered by the request. The browser might first question if this relatively small book fulfills a need, and second ask if it fulfills the need well. The answer to both questions is a resounding "Yes."

With the body of medical knowledge doubling every 5 years or so, the information that must either have been learned or be readily available and understandable to both the young as well as the experienced plastic surgeon continues to increase exponentially. This book distills present knowledge into an easily readable guide to almost any emergency a plastic surgeon might face who is on-call in the emergency room, or responding to a late night/early morning call from the hospital relating to a postoperative patient.

The authors, who are general plastic surgeons and specialists from the Division of Plastic Surgery here at the Baylor College of Medicine, have culled information from their own surgical experiences, as well as a wide variety of outside sources. They have condensed this knowledge into a small, handy volume, which could easily be read either at one's leisure or immediately prior to assuming the care of a patient. It would be difficult to find an injury or complication from a plastic surgery operation whose emergency treatment is not covered in this book. The authors have detailed the specifics in terms of differential diagnosis and the corrective steps necessary to fulfill the responsibilities of a plastic surgeon answering emergency room call.

There are many references to the general principles of treatments—those learned in residency training and in the early years of practice that have stood the test of time. The ability of the surgeon to present an organized treatment plan and then carry it out expeditiously will instill confidence in the patient and the health care personnel involved in the treatment of these patients. The format of the book is conducive to allowing readers to add both personal and technical notes, which will serve them well in the treatment of future patients with similar injuries.

I would be remiss if I didn't call special attention to the lead author, Dr. Jamal M. Bullocks, whose ability and youthful enthusiasm has amalgamated the thoughts and experience of the other authors into a volume that will find great value for all plastic surgeons as well as general surgeons and emergency room physicians.

To those older plastic surgeons who may believe that they have already learned the answers to most of the problems presenting to the plastic surgeon on call, I respectfully suggest that although the problems that presented a decade or two ago may be the same, the answers (i.e., treatment) today may be different. It is to that difference that we are indebted to the authors of this book for their effort and time in providing us with concise and practical answers.

Melvin Spira, M.D., D.D.S.
Division of Plastic Surgery
Department of Surgery
Baylor College of Medicine

Preface

Severe facial trauma, soft tissue and hand injuries, and the postoperative care of plastic surgery patients often present great challenges to the acute care physician. In addition, the method of treatment at the initial time of presentation often dictates the ultimate functional and cosmetic outcome for the patient. The rapid pace of activity in the emergency room or during an on-call night consultation can easily lead to a delay in patient diagnosis and treatment if extensive research is required on unfamiliar topics. *Plastic Surgery Emergencies* is designed to provide updated, easy-to-follow instructions and clear illustrations to optimize the effectiveness of treatment of patients with acute plastic surgery issues. This book, through its concisely outlined principles and procedures, will guide medical practitioners in their approach to the patient at this most critical time period.

We attempted to include all topics that we ourselves have faced while taking plastic surgery call at the affiliated hospitals in the Texas Medical Center, one of the largest medical centers in the world, which sees over 100,000 patients per day. The included topics are outlined with the information, tools, and pharmacotherapy needed for acute patient management. The chapters are designed in an outline format for rapid transfer of erudite and practical information. With more than 100 original drawings and photographs, *Plastic Surgery Emergencies*, we hope, will serve as a one-step, quick-reference source to aid in the efficient diagnosis and appropriate treatment of patients.

Whether used by a resident facing a congested flap, a rural physician facing a hand infection, or an emergency room physician facing a mangled extremity, *Plastic Surgery Emergencies* will provide in-depth, easy-to-follow directions that will allow optimized care for the patient and provide confidence for the practitioner.

♦ Acknowledgments

This volume would not be possible without the hard work, dedication, and patience of the faculty, residents, and staff (past and current) of the Division of Plastic Surgery in the Michael E. Debakey Department of Surgery at the Baylor College of Medicine and its affiliated hospitals in the Texas Medical Center.

Lastly, this book would not be complete without the skill and dedication of the illustrator, Mike de la Flor, and the cover artist, Cara Ryan Downey, MD.

List of Abbreviations

3D	three-dimensional
ABCs	airway, breathing, and circulation
AP	anteroposterior
b.i.d.	twice daily
BP	blood pressure
BSA	burned surface area
BSS	balanced saline solution
C-spine	cervical spine
CBC	complete blood count
CHEM-7	a basic metabolic panel
CMP	carpometacarpal
CRP	C-reactive protein
CSF	cerebrospinal fluid
CT	computed tomography
CVP	central venous pressure
CXR	chest X-ray
DIC	disseminated intravascular coagulation
DIP	distal interphalangeal
EMG	electromyogram
ENOG	electroneurography
ENT	ear, nose, and throat
ESR	erythrocyte sedimentation rate
FFP	fresh frozen plasma
IM	intramuscularly
INR	international normalized ratio
IP	interphalangeal
IV	intravenously
IV/PO	intravenously or orally
IVF	intravenous fluid

LR	lactated Ringer's
MAP	mean arterial pressure
MCP	metacarpophalangeal
MRI	magnetic resonance imaging
NCS	nerve conduction studies
NOE	naso-orbital-ethmoid
NPO	nothing by mouth
NS	normal saline
ORIF	open reduction, internal fixation
PIP	proximal interphalangeal
pRBC	packed red blood cells
PRN	as needed
PT	prothrombin time
PTT	partial thromboplastin time
q.d.	once daily
q.i.d.	four times daily
q12h	every 12 hours
q2h	every 2 hours
q6h	every 6 hours
q8h	every 8 hours
qAM	each morning
ROM	range of motion
RR	relative risk
SBP	systolic blood pressure
SC	subcutaneously
SSEP	somatosensory-evoked potential
STAT	at once, immediately
t.i.d.	three times daily
TBSA	total body surface area

1

Wound Management

♦ Evaluation

Before wound treatment is performed, a full evaluation of the wound must be undertaken.

Acute Wounds

1. Assess size, shape, and location
2. Determine the timing of the wound – acute (time elapsed since injury) versus chronic (persistent >3 months)
3. Establish laceration, avulsion, or chronic open wound
4. Evaluate the wound for odor, exudate, purulent drainage, bleeding, and debris
5. Determine if there is exposure of vessels, tendons, nerves, joint, muscle, or bone
6. Evaluate for foreign bodies in the wound: consider X-ray evaluation—if the history is inconsistent with clinical evaluation.

Chronic Wounds

Chronic wounds require investigation into reasons why proper wound healing is not accomplished.

Intrinsic Inhibitions of Wound Healing	Exogenous Inhibitions of Wound Healing

Poor blood supply
Infection
  Bacterial contamination
    >10^5 or 10^4 group B streptoccocus species
  Wound tension or pressure
    >30 mmHg
	Advanced age
	Malignancy
	Poor nutrition
	History of radiation
	Severe symptoms of disease (e.g., diabetes)
	Immunosuppression
	Smoking

Therefore, chronic contamination wounds warrant serologic evaluation to include

WBC
Hct/HbB
Albumin
Pre albumin, B transferin
ESR/SED

♦ Treatment

Acute Wounds

Irrigation in the acute wound setting is designed to remove blood, foreign bodies, debris, and bacteria from a wound. This can easily be accomplished with a 1-L bottle of normal saline with two or three holes punched into the cap with an 18-gauge needle. When squeezed forcefully, it serves as an effective pressurized irrigator. The wound should be irrigated until all visible debris is washed away. Anesthetizing the wound prior to irrigation and débridement provides for greater patient comfort and allows for aggressive decontamination of the wound.

Chronic Wounds

Simple surface irrigation of a chronic wound is usually only marginal and minimally effective. It can be useful at the bedside if there is debris grossly evident in the wound. Studies have shown that pressure irrigation at ~70 psi is needed to reduce bacteria count and particulate matter. This is best done in the operating room with a PulsaVac Wound Debridement System (Zimmer, Inc., Warsaw, IN) or a jet lavage system. If needed, a thorough débridement of devitalized tissue can also be done in the operating room.

♦ Débridement and Hemostasis

Adequate débridement of devitalized tissue and skin edges is important in preparing the contaminated wound for closure. The skin is highly vascular and excessive skin removal is usually not necessary. Jagged skin edges should be trimmed to facilitate an easier closure. Hemostasis is achieved with pressure, silver nitrate, fibrin, Surgicel (Johnson & Johnson, New Brunswick, NJ), thrombin, or suture ligature (absorbable for small vessels and nonabsorbable for larger vessels) to prevent hematoma formation. If there is any question as to the viability of the tissue, it is better to allow the tissue to demarcate rather than to débride it initially. Tissue of questionable viability can often undergo necrosis after débridement due to retrograde thrombosis. Once demarcated, the tissue can be débrided to healthy bleeding tissue.

♦ Closure and Antibiotics

Prior to closure, irrigation, débridement, hemostasis and trimming of the skin's jagged edges should be performed. A tension-free closure will help to ensure scar-free healing.

Most clean lacerations, if addressed in <8 hours, have minimal contamination and can be closed primarily without the need for antibiotics. Clean wounds presenting after 8 hours can be closed after débridement of the entire wound and sharp débridement of edges. This would include stab wounds, lacerations by window or glass, and clean avulsions. On the other hand, contaminated wounds, such as wounds with dirt and debris, should be treated with systemic antibiotics with additional consideration for tetanus prophylaxis.

Choice of antibiotics should usually cover gram-positive organisms (cefazolin 1 gm IV). Due to the increase in methicillin-resistant *Staphylococcus aureus* (MRSA), certain wounds may require other antibiotics for coverage (clindamycin 600 mg IV or vancomycin 1 g IV). The astute caregiver should take advantage of administration of a single IV dose of antibiotics to wounds at risk for contaminations while the patient is in a health care setting undergoing evaluation.

If the wound is grossly contaminated with debris or if the patient is a diabetic, broader spectrum antibiotics should be considered, for example, Avelox (Bristol-Myers Squibb, New York, NY) 400 mg IV/PO q.d., Zosyn (Wyeth Pharmaceuticals, Collegeville, PA) 3.375 g IV q6h, Imipinem (Merck, Sharp, & Dohme, Whitehouse Station, NJ) 1 g IV q8h, or combination therapy.

Contaminated wounds should be left open except for those on the face. Wet to dry dressing changes should be done at least twice a day. In addition, the patient should shower frequently and wash the wound with soap and water.

A 5- to 7-day course of outpatient antibiotics may also be warranted. Coverage should include gram-positive and MRSA coverage (clindamycin 450 mg PO q.i.d., Bactrim double strength (DS) PO b.i.d.) Cephalexin is not effective in treating a contaminated wound. Rarely, acute wounds will require inpatient treatment with IV antibiotics. Usually, though, débridement and prophylactic PO ABs should suffice. In the case of more subacute or chronic wounds with gross contamination or purulent considerations should be made for admission IV antibiotics and formal débridement.

Skin-Flap Wound Closure

If the patient has an avulsed skin flap, the flap should be tacked down where it lies (**Fig. 1–1**). *Do not put tension on the skin flap for complete closure*. Tension will lead to total flap loss. First, débride all devitalized tissue and then inset the flap so that no tension is present. Distal margins of the flap will usually necrose. Plan on redébridement as the flap demarcates.

Tetanus Prophylaxis

Tetanus-prone wounds are old (>6 hours), deep (>1 cm), and/or contaminated, especially those that involve rusty metal, feces, or soil. Depending on the degree of contamination, tetanus toxoid, tetanus immunoglobin or complete immunization may be required. Specific recommendations for tetanus prophylaxis are included in **Table 1–1**, **Table 1–2**, and **Table 1–3**.

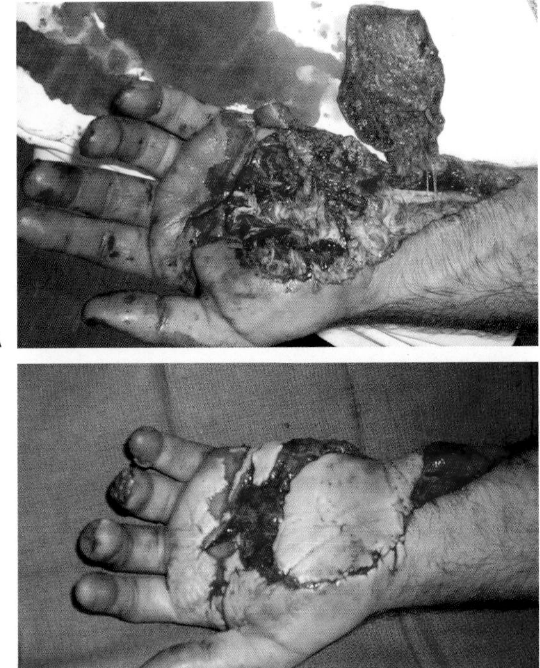

Figure 1–1 **(A)** Avulsed skin flap. **(B)** Avulsed skin flap taken down without tension

Table 1–1 Tetanus-Prone Wounds

Clean (Low Risk)	Tetanus Prone (High Risk)
Clean incised wound Superficial graze Scalded skin	Any wound or burn >6 h old Contact with soil, manure, or compost Puncture-type wound Infected wound Compound fracture Large amount of devitalized tissue Animal or human bite

Table 1–2 Immunization Status and Tetanus Risk

Immunization Status	Low Risk	Moderate Risk	High Risk
Fully immunized, <5 y since booster	None	None	None
Fully immunized, 5–10 y since booster	None	Td	Td
Fully immunized, >10 y since booster	Td	Td	Td + TIG
Incompletely immunized or uncertain	Full tetanus vaccine	Full tetanus vaccine + TIG	Full tetanus vaccine + TIG

Abbreviations: Td, tetanus toxoid; TIG, tetanus immunoglobulin.

Table 1–3 Recommendations for Vaccination with Tetanus Immunoglobulin

Patient	Dosage	Treatment
Adult	250–500 units	For both patient groups, the vaccine should be given IM in the opposite upper extremity (arm) to the tetanus toxoid
Pediatric	250 units	

♦ Follow-up

Careful and frequent follow-up is imperative for all wounds. Patients should be asked to return to the clinic or general practitioner within 3 days if possible and educated on all the signs and symptoms of an infection. Specific instructions on wound care and antibiotic therapy are crucial to guaranteeing patient compliance and ultimately a favorable prognosis.

2

Anesthesia and Wound Closure

All wounds should be clean of foreign bodies and adequately irrigated (see Chapter 1). Hemostasis is achieved with pressure, silver nitrate, fibrin, Surgicel (Johnson & Johnson, New Brunswick, NJ), thrombin, or suture ligature (absorbable for small vessels and nonabsorbable for larger vessels) to prevent hematoma formation. Any devitalized tissue as well as jagged edges should be trimmed for optimal cosmesis.

Wounds can be closed with sutures, staples, skin tapes, or wound adhesives. Generally, wounds should be closed in layers using appropriate sutures and the epidermis reapproximated relatively tension free and everted if possible. Everted skin edges eventually flatten out and produce a level wound surface where the inverted skin edge persists to produce a valley-like scar.

In order to guarantee a successful wound closure a comfortable environment should be created for both the practitioner and patient. The use of analgesics, local anesthesia, and—at times—sedation are helpful adjunct in reducing patient anxiety. This will ultimately increase the likelihood of more precise closure.

♦ Anesthesia

Local Anesthetics

Local anesthetics work by affecting the sodium (Na^+) channels on afferent sensory nerves. Local anesthetics enter the cell membranes and reversibly binding to the Na channels, the cells are then unable to depolarize. Lidocaine is probably the most commonly used and accessible local anesthetic agent in the emergency room (ER).

Epinephrine can be used along with lidocaine to decrease the amount of lidocaine needed, prolong the duration of the anesthetic, and decrease the amount of bleeding from the site (through vasoconstriction). The maximum safe dose for lidocaine is 4 mg/kg. With the addition of epinephrine (usually at 1:100,000 concentration), the maximum dose increases to 7 mg/kg.

A 1% solution of lidocaine is defined as

$$1\ g/100\ cc = 10\ g/1000\ cc = 10{,}000\ mg/1000\ cc = 10\ mg/1\ cc$$

Example Maximum dose of lidocaine with epinephrine in a 70-kg (154-lb) man

$$70\ kg \times \text{max dose}\ (7 mg/kg) = 490\ mg\ \text{of lidocaine}$$

$$490\ mg \times 1\ cc/10\ mg\ (\text{concentration of } 1\%\ \text{lidocaine}) = 49\ cc\ \text{of } 1\%\ \text{lidocaine with epinephrine}$$

Epinephrine should not be used near end arteries, including the penis, digits, the nose, or stellate lacerations to avoid ischemia and necrosis. Wait 7 to 15 minutes for the epinephrine to become effective. **Table 2–1** provides other local anesthetics that may be used with their maximum dosages and duration of action.

Once you have chosen your local anesthetic, it is useful to add bicarbonate to the solution, particularly when the patient is awake. The pH of local anesthetic solutions is generally buffered between 4 to 5 to prolong shelf life. Due to this acidity, patients often experience burning on injection. By adding a base to the local anesthetic, the action will also be accelerated because the higher pH favors the nonionized form of the anesthetic, which crosses the

Table 2–1 Local Anesthetics for Wound Closure

Drug	Onset	Maximum Dose mg/kg (with Epinephrine mg/kg)	Duration (with Epinephrine)
Lidocaine	Rapid	4.5 (7)	120 min (240 min)
Mepivacaine	Rapid	5 (7)	180 min (360 min)
Bupivacaine	Slow	2.5 (3)	4 h (8 h)
Procaine	Slow	8 (10)	45 min (90 min)
Chloroprocaine	Rapid	10 (15)	30 min (90 min)
Etidocaine	Rapid	2.5 (4)	4 h (8 h)
Prilocaine	Medium	5 (7.5)	90 min (360 min)
Tetracaine	Slow	1.5 (2.5)	3 h (10 h)

cell membrane more easily. The addition of 1 cc of a 1 mEq/mL solution of bicarbonate for every 9 cc of local anesthetic can alleviate this burning and improve patient comfort. Warming the anesthetic, using a 25-gauge needle or higher, and injecting by inserting the needle within the wound (instead of through the skin), helps in decreasing the pain felt by the patient on injection.

Topical Anesthetics

- *Eutectic mixture of local anesthetics (EMLAs)* 2.5% prilocaine and 2.5% lidocaine cream
- *Lidocaine-epinephrine-tetracaine (LET) gel* 4% lidocaine, 1:2000 epinephrine, 1% tetracaine

The duration and the depth of the blockade is dependent on the time the cream is in contact with the skin. Apply to the wound and then cover with a Tegaderm (3M, St. Paul, MN) or another occlusive dressing. The cream or gel will usually need to be in place for at least 45 minutes before *any* anesthetic effect is achieved.

Digital and Facial Nerve Blocks

Please see respective chapters for hand (Chapter 18) and face laceration (Chapter 8).

Conscious Sedation

Fear and anxiety is commonly encountered in the pediatric patient in the ER. Therefore, it may be difficult to suture a child's wound because, understandably, the patient may be uncooperative. Conscious sedation may be used if conditions are appropriate and the necessary precautions are followed. A well-trained pediatrician or anesthesiologist should be consulted for administration of conscious sedation, especially if the surgeon's experience is limited in this field. Full monitoring by a nurse is required throughout the procedure.

Prior to administering conscious sedation, a complete history and physical examination should be obtained, including

- age
- weight (measured, not estimated, whenever possible)
- vital signs

- oxygen saturation
- absence of head injury (document)
- heart, lung, neurological, and mental status
- size and location of injury and neurovascular status distal to it

Prior to sedation, there should be

- no oral liquids up to 2 hours prior to procedures in children <2 years of age – 3 hours if >3 years
- no milk or solid food for 8 hours prior to the procedure

During the procedure,

- maintain continuous oxygen saturation and heart rate monitoring
- record vital signs and blood pressure every 15 minutes for conscious sedation and every 5 minutes for deep sedation
- record drug dose and time administered
- record state of consciousness and response to stimulation

As precautionary measures, ensure that

- a nasal cannula and intubation tray are available during the procedure
- a reversal agent is ready and prepared in syringe (Narcan [DuPont Pharma, Wilmington, DE] 0.4 mg IV push q2 to 3 minutes PRN, flumazenil 0.2 mg IV push given over 30 seconds, then 0.3 mg IV push given over 30 seconds PRN, maximum total dose 3 mg)
- a suctioning apparatus and canister are available
- nursing staff is in the room during the procedure to assist
- drug combinations that include amnestic and analgesic effects are used

The common drugs used are as follows (**Table 2–2**):

- for adults:
  - short procedure: Versed (Hoffman LaRoche, Nutley, NJ) + fentanyl
  - moderate interval procedure: morphine + Ativan (Biovail Pharmaceuticals, Inc., Bridgewater, NJ)

Table 2–2 Conscious Sedation for Wound Closure

Drug	Description	Adult Dose	Pediatric Dose	Onset of Sedation
Fentanyl	Analgesic, sedative	0.5–1 g/kg/dose IV/IM every 30–60 min	2–10 g/kg IV/IM every 1–2 h	1–3 min (IV)
Versed	Sedative-hypnotic, amnestic	0.5–2 mg IV over 2–3 min	0.25–0.5 mg/kg PO/IM 0.05–0.1 mg/kg IV	15 min (IM) 2.5 min (IV)
Ativan	Sedative-hypnotic, amnestic	2 mg total or 0.044 mg/kg IV	0.05–0.1 mg/kg IV slowly over 2–5 min	1 h (IM) 15–20 min (IV)
Ketamine	Analgesic, amnestic	1–4.5 mg/kg IV 3–8 mg/kg IM	6–10 mg/kg PO once, 30 min prior to procedure 0.5–2 mg/kg IV once 3–7 mg/kg IM once	3–4 min (IM) 30 s (IV)
Propofol	Sedative-hypnotic, amnestic	3 mg/mg h (IV)	Not recommended for children under 16	40 s (IV)
Morphine	Analgesic, sedative	5–20 mg IM 2.5–15 mg IV over 4–5 min	0.1–0.2 mg/kg	15–30 min (IM) 5–10 min (IV)

- for pediatric patients:
  - ketamine + Versed

For all patients, start with a subtherapeutic dose, then re-bolus in small intervals to titrate sedative effect.

Sutures

A variety of suture material is available and in general, can be differentiated based on **(Table 2–3)**

- absorbable versus nonabsorbable
- braided versus nonbraided
- tensile strength half-life

Table 2–3 Suture Materials for Wound Closure

Suture Material	Absorbable vs. Nonabsorbable	Monofilament vs. Braided	Half-life	Strength Profile	Absorption Profile	Common Uses
Plain gut	Absorbable	Monofilament	7–10 d	75% at 7 d	2 mo	Pediatric skin closure
Chromic	Absorbable	Monofilament	2 wk	12% at 14 d	3 mo	Mucosal closure
Vicryl	Absorbable	Braided	2–3 wk	65% at 2 wk 8% at 4 wk	2 mo	Deep dermal muscle fascia
PDS	Absorbable	Monofilament	4 wk	70% at 3 wk 25% at 6 wk	6–8 mo	Muscle fascia
Monocryl	Absorbable	Monofilament	1–2 wk	50% at 1 wk 20% at 2 wk	3–4 mo	Deep dermal, subcuticular
Silk	Nonabsorbable	Braided	Permanent	-	-	Bolsters hemostasis
Nylon	Nonabsorbable	Monofilament	Permanent	-	-	Skin
Prolene	Nonabsorbable	Monofilament	Permanent	-	-	Skin tendon

Abbreviations: PDS, polydioxanone suture.

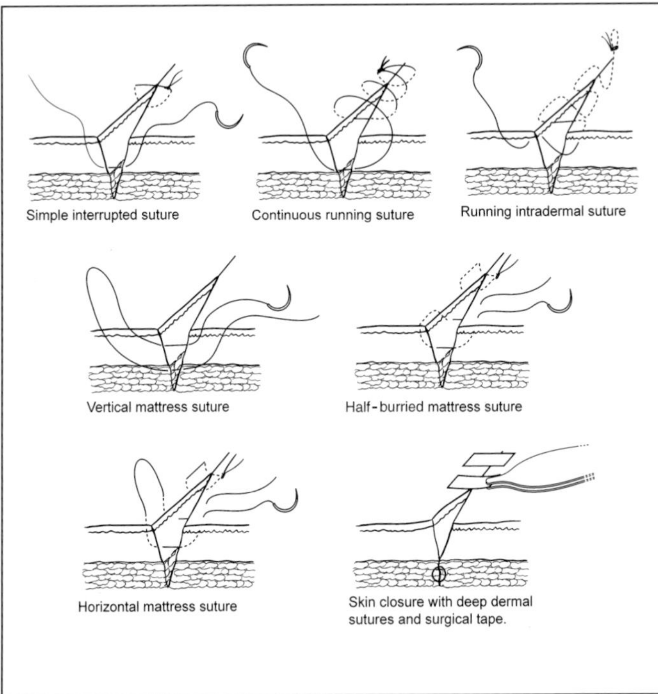

Figure 2–1 Suture techniques.

The types of needle that are available in the ER are the

- Taper/round needle: Use in muscle and cartilage and mucosa
- Cutting needle: For skin
  - Use a half-circle cutting needle for subcutaneous tissue
  - Use a 3/8-circle cutting needle for skin

Suture techniques include (**Fig. 2–1**)

- *Simple interrupted* general tissue approximation
- *Simple running* fast and effective for long lacerations. The entire suture must be removed should infection ensue.
- *Vertical mattress* most effective in everting skin edges. However, it may cause skin necrosis.

- *Horizontal mattress* effective in everting skin edges. However, it may cause skin necrosis.
- *Running subcuticular* closing skin suture for clean wounds in the operating room
- *Staples* a fast procedure and usually used on the scalp or dirty wound that is closed loosely. The staples should be removed in 5 days to avoid epithelization and a poor cosmetic result.
- *Adhesive skin tape* can be used to reapproximate small lacerations with very little tension
- *Dermabond* skin adhesive that can be used for clean lacerations with no jagged edges. After the wound is adequately prepared, reapproximate skin edges with a finger and apply the first coat, let it dry for 20 seconds, then apply a second coat. (Care must be taken to prevent any foreign materials from entering the wound.)

In conclusion, the astute practitioner will first anesthetize the patient's wound, débride it meticulously with removal of jagged edges, and close the would with care to reapproximate the dermal and epidermal layers of the skin, to provide the patient the greatest chance of recovery without infection and the best cosmetic result.)

3

Pressure Sores

The treatment of pressure sores is often one of the most difficult challenges of plastic surgery. Commonly, patients with pressure sores present acutely with signs of systemic infection. Pressure sores are a chronic problem in sedentary patients with multiple systemic problems. Thus it is essential to keep in mind that the likely source of acute systemic infection is not the sore itself. Each case warrants a complete evaluation by the examiner to rule out the pressure sore as the likely cause of the infection.

♦ Pressure Sore Staging System (Fig. 3–1)

Stage 1 Intact skin with nonblanchable erythema

Stage 2 Superficial ulcer involving partial thickness of the epidermis and dermis; usually presents as an abrasion, blister, or very shallow ulcer

Stage 3 Full-thickness skin loss down to the subcutaneous tissue, which does not extend beyond underlying fascia

Stage 4 Full-thickness skin loss down through subcutaneous tissue with involvement of muscle, bone, tendon, ligament, or joint capsule

♦ Evaluation

- Position the patient in a well-lighted area to facilitate visualization of the ulcer.
- Gently probe the wound and assess for fluid collections or purulent drainage. If pus is present, incision and drainage (I&D)

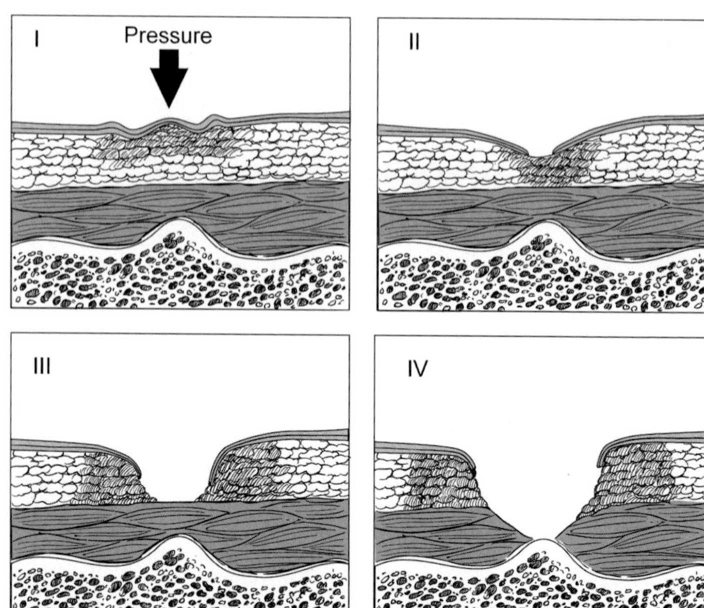

Figure 3–1 Pressure sore staging system.

should be performed and the wound irrigated copiously and packed wet to dry (see below). Obtain a culture and samples of the purulent material.

- Necrotic soft tissue is common. If it is devoid of purulent drainage, it is unlikely to be the source of sepsis. Copious drainage may be indicative of a much larger wound beneath the skin.
- Subcutaneous fat and muscle are more prone to ischemia than skin. Therefore, intact skin (possibly with small eschar) may harbor a large area of necrotic tissue below making the wound unstageable. Often, an eschar at or above the adjacent skin layer is indicative of partial skin thickness loss. An eschar that is depressed may represent full-thickness skin loss.
- Radiographically assess the area to determine the presence of underlying deep soft tissue (CT scan) or bony infection (X-ray).
- Check available studies – CBC, blood cultures, CXR, blood sugar, albumin and pre-albumin, ESR, C-RP, and urinalysis.

- Rule out other possible systemic causes of fever – pneumonia, central lines, and urinary tract infections.
- Check for incontinence.

♦ Treatment

General treatment for all ulcers includes

- alleviation of pressure – place patient on an air-fluid mattress; use pillows, egg cartons, donuts
- avoidance of sheering forces
- frequent turning of the patient, q2h
- cleaning away incontinence – use a Foley catheter or a rectal tube (a maximum 24 hours)
- maximizing nutrition (albumin >3.0, prealbumin >18)

For staged ulcers:

- *Stage 1* Use moisturizers to prevent dryness.
- *Stage 2* No débridement is necessary; use occlusive dressings such as polyurethane film (Duoderm) or hydrocolloids.
- *Stages 3 and 4* Sharp débridement is often necessary with the addition of pulse lavage irrigation. Wounds are packed wet to dry with Kerlix. (Kendall Co., Mansfield, MA)

All ulcers should be débrided adequately of necrotic tissue; however, this is usually done in the operating room because of pain and the potential for uncontrolled bleeding. Minimal necrotic tissue can often be débrided at bedside with a local anesthesia, scissors, and a scalpel. If the patient is paraplegic, anesthetic may not be necessary. However, good hemostasis must be attained. Wet to dry dressings are done with normal saline (or 0.25% Dakin's solution) and Kerlix to débride the wound. First, wet the tip of the Kerlix and place it in the wound. Do not place wet Kerlix on the skin; this will eventually cause maceration of the skin. The dressing should be changed q8h. Dakin's 0.25% or acetic acid 0.25% solution can be used on the purulent wound; however, it should be discontinued once the wound is clean to avoid tissue destruction. Ask the hospital's wound care team to lavage the wound daily and continue débridement. Avoid placing tape on the skin. Duoderm may be placed on either side of the wound, thereby avoiding frequent tape contact directly with the skin.

If the patient is seen in the emergency room and there is no cellulitis, no elevation in white blood cell count, and no purulent drainage, then the wound can be débrided as necessary and the patient can be seen as an outpatient. In these cases, instruct the family on (1) dressing changes every 8 hours, (2) the importance of keeping the wound clean, and (3) the need for frequent turning of the patient. If the patient presents with cellulitis and purulent drainage of the wound, then admission to the hospital should be considered, especially if the patient has comorbid conditions.

Silvadene (Sanofi-Aventis Pharmaceuticals, Paris, France), or sulfamylon, can be used in selective cases of wounds with eschars. In an attempt to decolonize the wound surface temporalily, definitive débridement is undertaken. Betadyne swabs of the eschars are also useful in drying the wound to allow healing without further maceration. Culture swabs are of little use because all wounds are colonized, even the clean granulating wound. A quantitative tissue biopsy can be obtained to evaluate tissue bacterial counts ($>10^5$ per gram of tissue), and bone biopsy to related osteomyelitis.

4

Bite Wounds

Although often treated by the emergency room (ER) physician, bite wounds are also treatment issues for the plastic surgeon because they often occur on the hands and face or can be the cause of significant soft tissue destruction on the body.

- Irrigate all wounds copiously with NS
- Débride devitalized tissue
- Drain any fluid collections
- Determine if tetanus prophylaxis is indicated
- Leave all wounds open except those on the face
- Evaluate the need for antibiotics

♦ Bites

Human

Human mouths contain some of the most concentrated and varied bacteria. Organisms include *Eikenella*, *Staphylococcus*, *Streptococcus viridans*, and *Bacteroides*. The general principles of contaminated wound management apply to all human bite wounds as mentioned above. In the acute bite, the wound must be assessed fully and irrigated copiously. The patient should be placed on appropriate prophylactic antibiotics and followed closely for any signs of infection.

The initial injury often appears minor to the patient; thus no care is sought until an infection develops. It is important to fully assess the patient in the ER and advise on hospital admission, IV antibiotics, and possible operative management when necessary.

Bite injuries require careful evaluation for a deep infection because of the relatively benign presentation of their appearance. At times, due to the close proximity of the skin and underlying structures, nerve and tendon injuries may also be present. Also, due to the inherent depth penetration by the tooth or fang, microorganisms easily seed the depth of wounds, allowing rapid dissemination along the deep planes of the fascia and subcutaneous tissue. Therefore, rule out a deep injury even when the presentation is a minor wound such as an abrasion.

- Evaluate wound for depth, foreign body, drainage, cellulitis
- Assess for crepitus (subcutaneous emphysema; C + S), which would indicate gas-forming organisms along the deep planes
- I + D and irrigate
- Pack wound
- Treat with antibiotics

Closed-Fist Injury (Fight Bite)

With closed-fist injuries, the force of the blow to the mouth will often break the skin enough to lacerate or infect the extensor tendon and contaminate the underlying joint, such as the metacarpophalangeal joint, with bacteria from the mouth. When the hand is placed back into a neutral position, the bacteria can be displaced, resulting in more proximal contamination. Aggressive irrigation and débridement in the operating room should be considered for grossly contaminated wounds and those that present late.

- Obtain hand series (rule out metacarpal head fracture, osteomyelitis, and dental foreign body)
- Evaluate the integrity of the extensor and flexor tendons (flexor tenosynovitis)
- Analyze purulent drainage (culture and sensitivities)
- Assess for crepitus
- Assess for loss of joint height, which would indicate metacarpal head fracture
- Irrigate site (if a joint is involved, irrigation in an operating room may be required)
- Treat with antibiotics

Antibiotics

First Line Augmentin (GlaxoSmithKline, Mississauga, Ontario, Canada)

Adult: 875 mg PO b.i.d. × 7 days

Pediatric: 45 kg/day PO b.i.d. × 7 days

Alternatives Unasyn 1.5 g IV q6h (Pfizer Pharmaceuticals, New York, NY)

Moxifloxacin 400 mg PO q.d. × 7 days

Clindamycin 450 mg PO q.i.d. + Bactrim (Roche Pharmaceuticals, Nutley, NJ) DS PO b.i.d. × 7 days

Cat

Cat bites are deeply penetrating wounds that are heavily contaminated, and approximately 80% of wounds become infected. Organisms include *Pasteurella multocida* and *Staphylococcus* species. Irrigate heavily, wash daily, treat with antibiotics, and see below for rabies vaccinatation criteria. Evaluate for tetanus prophylaxis. Do not close the wound.

Antibiotics

First Line Augmentin

Adult: 875 mg PO b.i.d. × 7 days

Pediatric: 45 kg/day PO b.i.d. × 7 days

Alternatives Doxycycline 100 mg PO b.i.d. × 7 days

Cefuroxime 0.5 g PO b.i.d. × 7 days

Dog

Dog bites constitute 80 to 90% of all animal bites. Organisms include *Pasteurella multocida*, *Bacteroides*, *Streptococcus viridans*, *Fusobacterium*, and *Capnocytophaga*. Massive force can often cause significant avulsion injuries; however, due to the lower bacterial count, infection is not seen as frequently as in cats. Large avulsion injuries can be reapproximated loosely as long as the wound can be packed and allowed to drain should an infection ensue. Elevate and treat with antibiotics. See below for rabies vaccination criteria. Evaluate for tetanus prophylaxis.

Antibiotics

First Line Augmentin
Adult: 875 mg PO b.i.d. × 7 days
Pediatric: 45 kg/day PO b.i.d. × 7 days
Alternative Unasyn 1.5 g IV q6h
Clindamycin 450 mg PO q.i.d. + Bactrim DS PO b.i.d. × 7 days

Rabies

Rabies is a viral infection of the central and peripheral nervous system that causes encephalitis with or without paralysis. If left untreated, it has close to 100% mortality. In the United States, rabies is most common in bats, raccoons, skunks, foxes, coyotes, ferrets, cats, and dogs. Bats are the most common wild animal to carry rabies. Cats are the most common domestic animals to carry rabies because of the high number of unvaccinated strays and their contact with raccoons, bats, and other wild animals.

Transmission is through the mucous membranes and saliva through breaks in the skin. The virus then replicates locally in the muscle and eventually travels through peripheral nerves to the spinal cord, then to the brain. Incubation times have ranged from as short as 5 days to as long as 7 years; however, the average incubation time is ~1 to 3 months.

The most common symptoms of rabies include

- paresthesias at the site of the bite
- hypersalivation
- hydrophobia
- altered mental status
- anxiety
- hyperactivity
- bizarre behaviors
- hypertension
- hyperthermia
- hyperventilation
- spasms and contractions of the neck muscles
- pharyngeal and respiratory muscle paralysis
- seizures

The wound should be copiously irrigated with normal saline. Devitalized tissue should be adequately débrided with all wounds left open to heal by secondary intention. Tetanus status should be determined and vaccine administered if indicated (see Chapter 1). A broad-spectrum antibiotic may be administered for 7 to 10 days (Augmentin 875 mg PO b.i.d.).

Domestic Animals

If the domestic animal's (e.g., cat, dog, ferret) rabies status is unknown, the animal should be quarantined and observed for 10 days; prophylaxis can be postponed if suspicion is relatively low. If the animal is rabid or if the presence of rabies is highly suspected, human rabies immune globulin (RIG) and human diploid cell rabies vaccine (HDCV) should be administered.

RIG = 20 IU/kg – 50% into the wound and 50% given IM

HDCV = given on days 0, 3, 7, 14, and 28

Wild Animals

Regard all wild animals (e.g., bats, foxes, coyotes, raccoons, skunks) as rabid. Test the animal if captured and administer RIG and HDCV to all patients as indicated above.

Snake

The majority of snakes are nonvenomous; however, the identification of the snake's species is imperative (**Fig. 4–1**).

History

- Time of bite
- Description of the snake
- Assess the timing of events and onset of symptoms. (Early and intense pain implies significant envenomation.)

Assessment

- Fang marks
- Edema
- Bullae

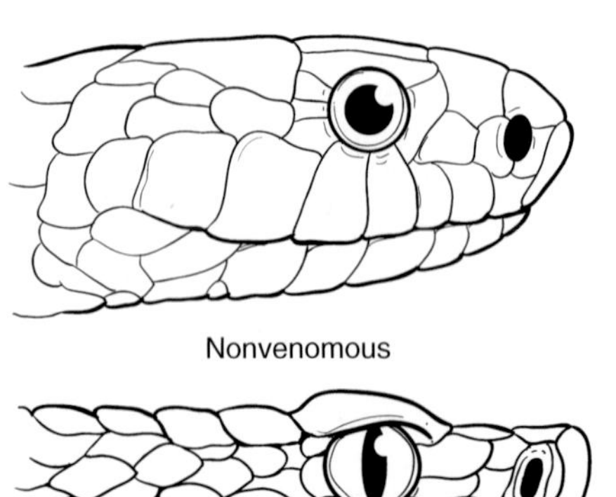

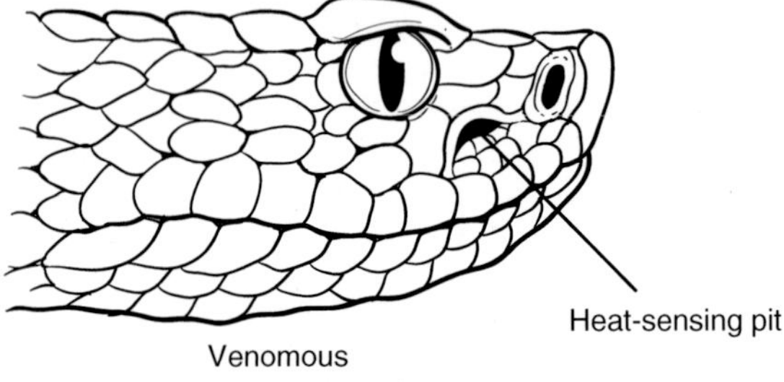

Fig. 4–1 Venomous versus nonvenomous snakes.

- Erythema
- Necrosis
- Crepitus
- Compartment syndrome
- Petechiae
- Paraesthesia
- Hemoptysis
- PT/PTT

Treatment

1. Immobilization, neutral positioning (splint) of extremity, and supportive care until transport to hospital. Suction devices on the bite can be effective in the first 15 to 30 minutes. Do not attempt incision over the bite, mouth suctioning, tourniquets, or ice packs.
2. Review the ABCs and evaluate the patient for signs of shock (e.g., tachypnea, tachycardia, dry pale skin, mental status changes, hypotension).

3. Obtain baseline laboratories including PT, PTT, INR, CXR, type and cross-match patient for FFP and pRBC.
4. Grading of envenomation
   - *Mild envenomation* local pain, edema, no signs of systemic toxicity, and normal laboratory values
   - *Moderate envenomation* severe local pain; edema larger than 12 inches surrounding the wound; and systemic toxicity including nausea, vomiting, and alterations in laboratory values (e.g., fallen hematocrit, or platelet values)
   - *Severe envenomation* characterized by generalized petechiae, ecchymosis, blood-tinged sputum, hypotension, hypoperfusion, renal dysfunction, changes in PT and activated PTT, and other abnormal tests defining consumptive coagulopathy
5. Antivenom is given for severe cases of snake envenomation. Serum sickness is possible with antivenoms, which are made with horse or sheep serum venom. A test dose is recommended; watch for an anaphylaxis reaction, which occurs in 1 to 39% of cases. Serum sickness is not an issue when snake antivenoms produced from recombinant DNA are used. Bites that are seen after 12 hours from initial injury usually do not need antivenom treatment if no systemic symptoms are present.

   Antivenom is given in ampules. One should start with 5 to 10 vials and continue therapy for up to 24 hours from the initial bite. If the patient responds (both a decrease in local and systemic reaction) to the antivenom, then depending on the antivenom used, a dosing regimen of antivenom is indicated. If the patient responds partially, plan to re-dose the antivenom. Ovine (sheep-derived) antivenin is also available. Allergic reaction to ovine antivenin recently has been reported. Patients should be monitored in an ICU setting during administration of antivenin for signs of allergic reaction.

   Coral snake bites ("red on yellow kill a fellow") are treated with antivenom, regardless of local or systemic signs, if the patient presents within 12 hours of bite. Coral snake bites can cause respiratory depression and alteration in the central nervous system – start with five vials of antivenom.
6. Evaluate the patient for compartment syndrome. If the patient begins to exhibit signs and symptoms of compartment syndrome (Chapter 19), immediate surgical intervention is indicated (fasciotomy).
7. Tetanus prophylaxis is indicated (Chapter 1).

8. Prophylactic antibiotic use is controversial; however, some recommendations include the following:
   - Rocephin 1 g IV q12h (Roche Pharmaceuticals, Nutley, NJ), or
   - Timentin 3.1 g IV q6h (GlaxoSmithKline, Mississauga, Ontario, Canada)
9. Elevate the involved extremity. This may require the aid of an IV pole, in which the extremity is hung using a stockinette.

Spider

There are over 20,000 species of spiders on earth. Dangerous species often encountered in North America include the brown recluse, black widow, hobo or aggressive house spider, and the yellow sac spider. Of these, only the brown recluse and the black widow have ever been associated with significant disease (**Fig. 4–2**).

The Brown Recluse Spider

The brown recluse spider has six eyes, a violin-shaped pattern on its thorax, and is found almost exclusively in the Midwestern and

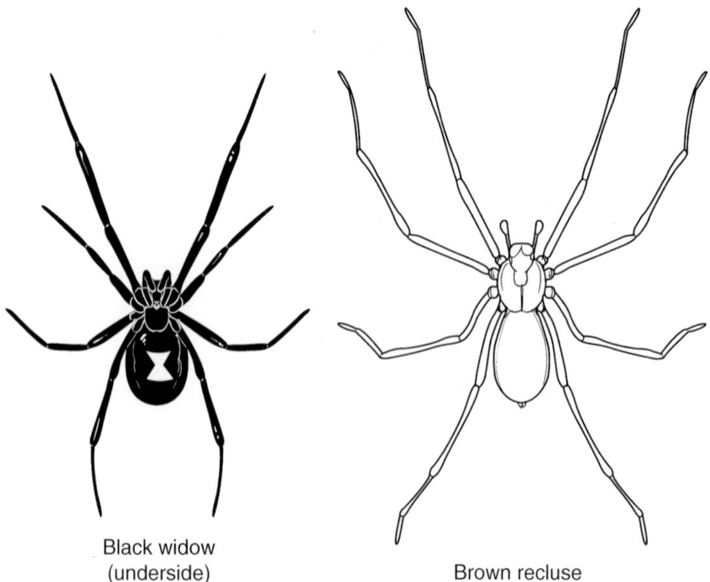

Fig. 4–2 The black widow and brown recluse spiders.

Southeastern states. Although the venom is more toxic than that of the rattlesnake, morbidity is usually not as severe because of the small amount of venom that can actually be injected by the creature. One of the specific enzymes in the venom causes destruction of skin, fat, and blood vessels. This process eventually leads to soft tissue necrosis at the site of the bite.

The venom also has a profound effect on the immune response, triggering the release of various inflammatory cytokines, histamines, and interleukins that can themselves cause further injuries and systemic responses. Although rare, these include

- destruction of red blood cells
- low platelet count
- blood clots in capillaries and loss of the ability to form clots where needed
- acute renal failure (kidney damage)
- coma
- death

One should carefully assess the patient for any of the above symptoms and admission is warranted for anyone exhibiting systemic toxicity. Apply ice to decrease pain and swelling, and elevate the site of injury above the heart. Wash the area thoroughly with soap and water and avoid any strenuous activity; this can facilitate the spread of the venom. Do not place heat on the area; this can accelerate tissue destruction. Do not attempt to suction the venom out and the use of steroid creams is not advised.

Brown recluse spider bites are usually painless at first and are slow to develop symptoms. Pain will usually present around 4 hours after the initial bite, with the bite wound presenting with a bulls-eye appearance. Blistering is then commonly seen 12 to 24 hours later with soft tissue necrosis to follow. Early débridement is not indicated and necrotic lesions should be kept clean and carefully dressed until spreading stops and the area of necrosis is well defined. A wide area of tissue around the skin can then be removed with subsequent skin grafting as needed.

- Baseline laboratories should include CBC, Chem-7, PT, PTT, INR
- There is no antivenom available; however, Dapsone 100 mg PO q.d. can be reserved for people with severe systemic disease (anemia, DIC, acute renal failure)

- Acetaminophen 325 mg, 1 to 2 tablets q4h, for pain. Avoid aspirin, ibuprofen (Motrin [Pfizer Pharmaceuticals, New York, NY], Advil [Wyeth Pharmaceuticals, Collegeville, PA], and naproxen (Aleve [Bayer Consumer Care, Morristown, NJ]).
- Benadryl 25 to 50 mg PO q6h PRN
- Antibiotics should be administered if significant soft tissue necrosis ensues.
- Patients should be watched very closely with follow-up the next day if possible.

The Black Widow Spider

Black widow spiders are nocturnal and are found in the Southern states. This spider has a distinctive red-colored hourglass figure on its underbelly. Its initial bite is usually associated with local pain followed by systemic reactions that can carry mortality as high as 5% (usually in children or the elderly). Generalized symptoms usually include

- nausea, vomiting
- faintness, dizziness
- chest pain
- hypotension
- tachycardia
- respiratory difficulties
- abdominal pain mimicking gallbladder or appendicitis

There is minimal tissue toxicity and the wound should be irrigated and cared for in the usual manor. Treatment for systemic symptoms is supportive and an antivenom is available for severe cases. It should only be used if the patient is unstable; usually, antivenom is not needed.

Cold compresses have been used to ease the pain at the site as well as over-the-counter pain medications. Over-the-counter pain medications can be used (e.g., Tylenol, naproxen, ibuprofen, Advil) as well as Benadryl (Pfizer Pharmaceuticals, New York, NY) 25 to 50 mg PO q6h for itching. In general, antibiotic prophylaxis and extensive medical follow-up is not needed.

5

Burns and Frostbite

Evaluation and management of the acutely burned patient is a common requirement of the plastic surgeon on-call. Rapid assessment, stabilization, and triage are essential for decreasing morbidity and mortality associated with burn injury. Commonly, the initial interview will be subsequent to the evaluation performed by the emergency room personnel. It is imperative, however, to remember to initiate measures to stop the burning process and practice universal safety precautions to confer increased safety for both the patient and the caregiver. If a child is burned and the mechanism of injury does not fit the burn pattern or if the patient was burned under unlikely circumstances or conditions, consider abuse.

♦ Burns

Initial Assessment – The ABCs

Airway

- Establish a patent airway via manual (chin lift, jaw thrust) or surgical techniques (cricoidectomy, tracheostomy)
- Assess for inhalational injury: signs and symptoms include soot deposits in the oropharynx, carbonaceous sputum, singed nasal hair, facial edema, hoarseness; determine whether the burns occurred while the patient was in an enclosed space

Table 5–1 The Glasgow Coma Scale (Score = $E + M + V$)

Eye opening (*E*)	
Spontaneous	4
To speech	3
To pain	2
No response	1
Best motor response (*M*)	
Obeys verbal command	6
Localizes painful stimulus	5
Flexion: withdrawal	4
Flexion: abnormal	3
Extension	2
No response	1
Best verbal response (*V*)	
Converses and oriented	5
Converses but disoriented	4
Inappropriate words	3
Incomprehensible sounds	2
No response	1

- Measure carboxyhemoglobin level: >10% requires oxygen therapy and is highly suggestive of an inhalation injury that requires intubation
- General criterion for intubation:
  - Glasgow Coma Score <8 (**Table 5–1**)
  - Inhalation injury
  - Deep facial and neck burns
  - Facial burns with associated TBSA burns >40%
  - Large TBSA burns – to allow adequate resuscitation
  - Oxygenation or ventilation compromise
    - PaO_2 <60
    - P_{CO2} >50
    - RR >40

Breathing

- Provide humidified oxygen by facemask
- Expose chest to assess ventilatory exchange, chest excursion, degree of chest wall injury, and presence of circumferential burns to the thorax
- Consider thoracic escharotomy for deep injury to the chest with associated ventilatory compromise

Circulation

- Establish vascular access with large-bore, high-flow venous cannulation. Avoid injured area if possible.
- Initiate monitoring: BP, pulse, temperature
- Consider invasive arterial lines for monitoring and frequent laboratory blood draws

Disability

- Gross assessment of neurological status (mnemonic tool = AVPU)
  Alert
  Responds only to Vocal painful stimuli
  Responds only to Painful stimuli
  Unresponsive to all stimuli
- Glasgow Coma Scale (**Table 5–1**)

Exposure

- Remove all clothing and debris to assess for gross injuries and for burn severity
- Prevent hypothermia by increasing the room temperature, covering the patient with clean warm linens, and infusing warm IV fluids

Burn Severity Assessment

For initial acute resuscitation, the following information is necessary:

- Height, weight, and age of the patient
- Depth of the burn injury; whether the burns are second or third degree
- Percentage of the total body surface area burned

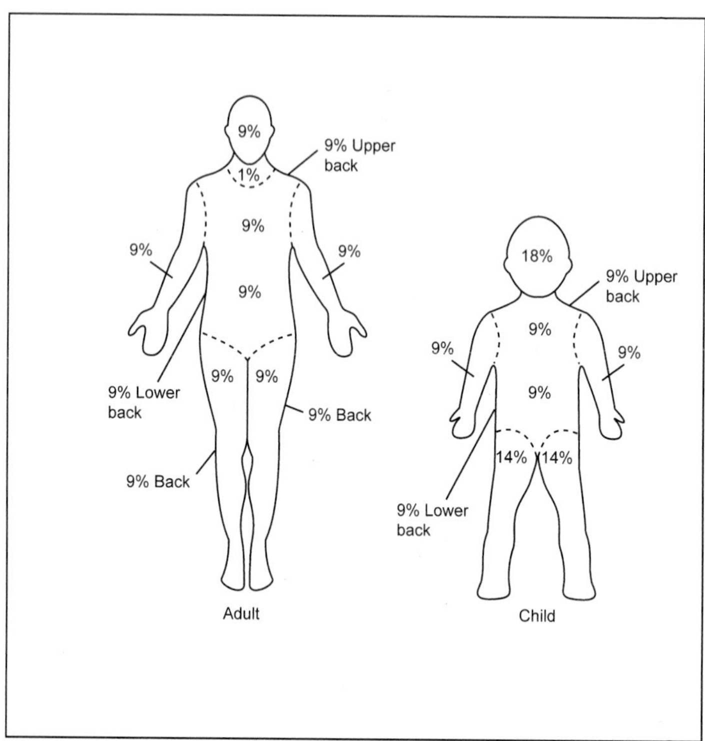

Figure 5–1 The "rule of nines" for adults and children.

The percentage of total body surface area (TBSA) can be estimated by the "rule of nines" (**Fig. 5–1**), or more accurately with burn charts (**Table 5–2**). Generally, the patient's hand (palm and fingers) is estimated as 1% of their total body surface area. The Burn Wound Classification is illustrated in **Fig. 5–2**.

Table 5–2 Lund and Browder Burn Estimate: Age versus Area

Area	Birth-1 year	1–4 years	5–9 years	10–14 years	15 years	Adult	2°	3°	TBSA %
Head	19	17	13	11	9	7			
Neck	2	2	2	2	2	2			
Anterior trunk	13	13	13	13	13	13			
Posteriortrunk	13	13	13	13	13	13			
Right buttock	2.5	2.5	2.5	2.5	2.5	2.5			
Left buttock	2.5	2.5	2.5	2.5	2.5	2.5			
Genitalia	1	1	1	1	1	1			
Right upper arm	4	4	4	4	4	4			
Left upper arm	4	4	4	4	4	4			
Right lower arm	3	3	3	3	3	3			
Left lower arm	3	3	3	3	3	3			
Right hand	2.5	2.5	2.5	2.5	2.5	2.5			
Left hand	2.5	2.5	2.5	2.5	2.5	2.5			
Right thigh	5.5	6.5	8	8.5	9	9.5			
Left thigh	5.5	6.5	8	8.5	9	9.5			
Right leg	5	5	5.5	6	6.5	7			
Left leg	5	5	5.5	6	6.5	7			
Right foot	3.5	3.5	3.5	3.5	3.5	3.5			
Left foot	3.5	3.5	3.5	3.5	3.5	3.5			
Total	100	100	100	100	100	100			

Epidermal Burns, First Degree (Fig. 5–3)

- Zones of injury are confined to the epidermis.
- Similar to sunburn
- Nonblanching erythema
- Very painful
- Heals in one week
- No significant scarring

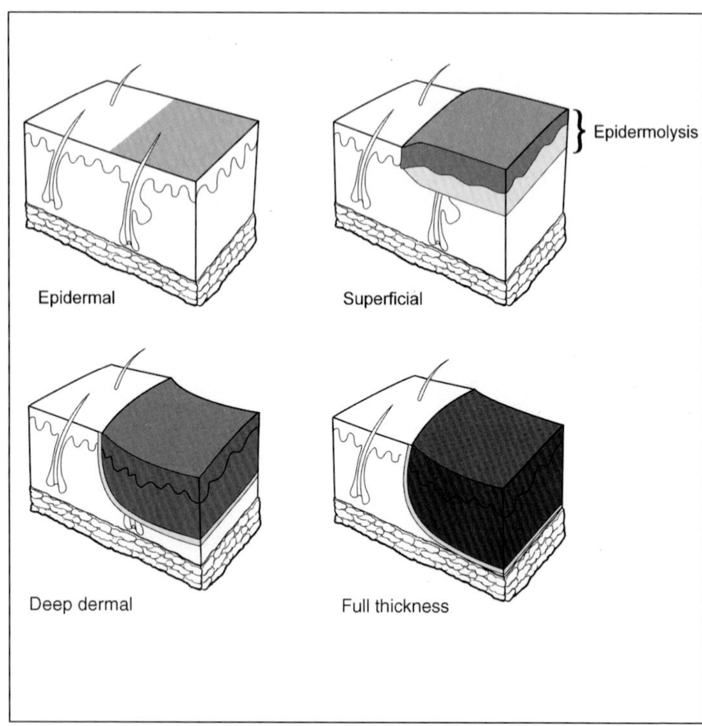

Figure 5–2 Burn wound classification.

Partial-Thickness Burns, Superficial Second Degree (Fig. 5–4)

- Confined to the upper third of the dermis
- The edema layer between the injured layer and normal dermis causes blistering.
- Commonly, these are the result of brief hot-liquid exposure.
- Wounds are wet, pink, and blistering.
- Wounds heal in 10 to 14 days with minimal scarring.

Partial-Thickness Burns, Mid-dermal Second Degree (Fig. 5–5)

- Result from longer hot-liquid exposure, grease, and flash flames
- Wounds are red, with minimal exudates and moderately painful.
- Wounds heal in 2 to 4 weeks with moderate scarring.

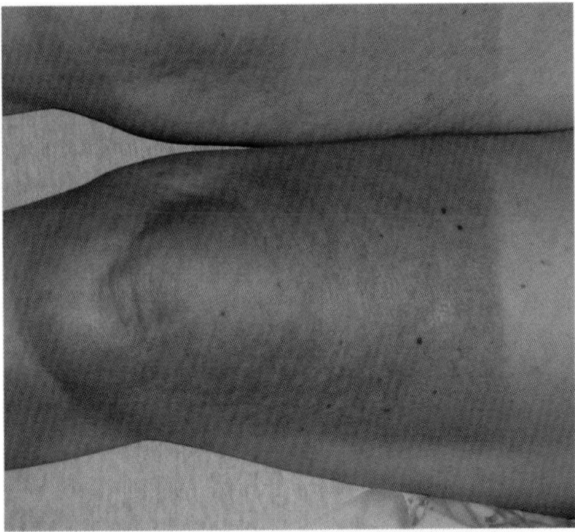

Figure 5–3 First-degree epidermal burn.

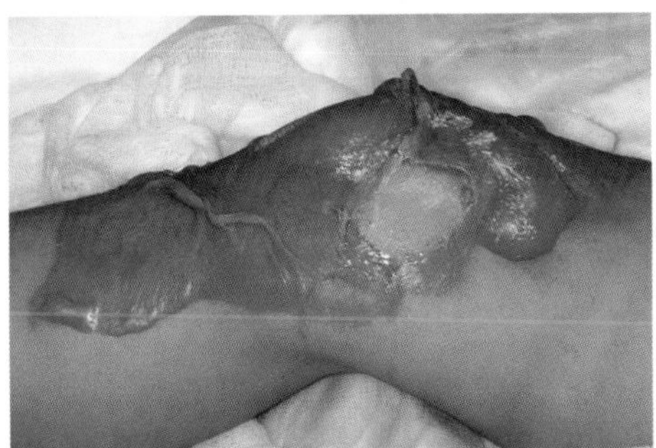

Figure 5–4 Superficial second-degree burn with blistering and epidermolysis.

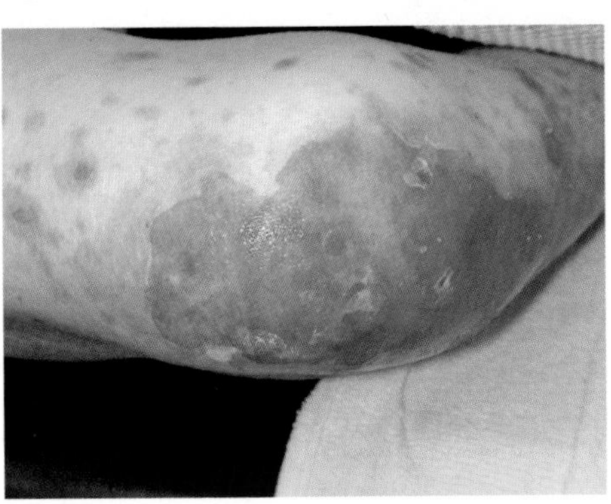

Figure 5–5 Mid-dermal second-degree burn.

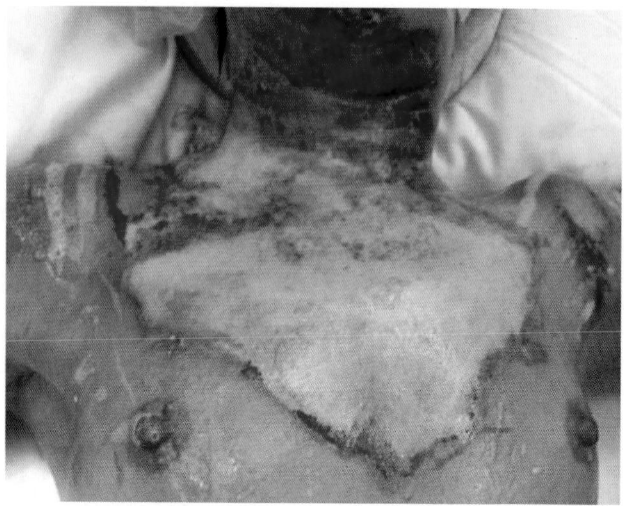

Figure 5–6 Deep-dermal third-degree burn with areas of full-thickness involvement.

Partial-Thickness Burns, Deep Dermal Third Degree (Fig. 5–6)

- Result from exposure to flames, grease, chemicals, and electricity
- Wounds are usually dry, white, and minimally painful (due to damage to nerve endings)
- Generally, wounds heal in 3 to 8 weeks with severe hypertrophic scarring.
- Excision and grafting will accelerate closure.

Full-Thickness Burns, Third Degree (Fig. 5–7)

- Result from high energy, and prolonged thermal exposure (chemicals, flames, electricity, explosions)
- Wounds are dry, white, or exhibit immediate eschar formation.
- Wounds are painless and insensate.
- These wounds need debridement and grafting to promote healing.

Burn Patient Resuscitation

Patients who require intravenous crystalloid resuscitation and possibly fluid balance monitoring with a Foley catheter placement are

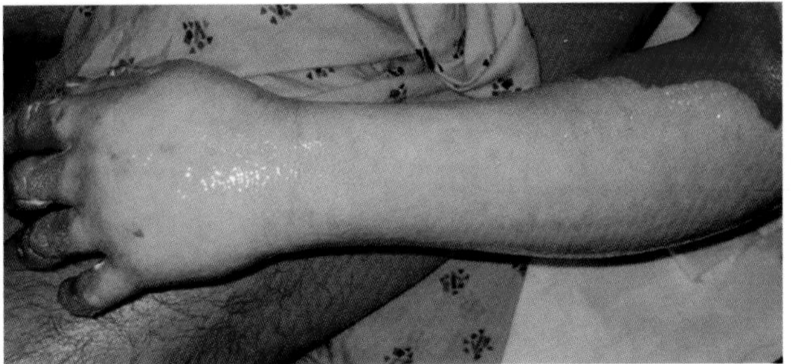

Figure 5–7 Full-thickness burn.

- adults with second and third degree burns >20% TBSA
- children (<14 years of age) with burns >15% TBSA
- infants (<2 years of age) with burns >10% TBSA

All other patients can be managed with oral hydration.

Urine output is used to gauge the success of fluid resuscitation. If there is any question as to the patient's ability to pass urine, place a Foley catheter. Lactated Ringer's solution should be started as soon as possible after the time of the burn. The volume of fluid given in the first 24 hours for adult victims is determined by the Parkland Formula:

$$4 \times \text{weight (kg)} \times \%\ \text{BSA} = \text{volume of fluid for 24 hours}$$

These estimates are based on second- and third-degree burn injuries only.

Pediatric patients have increased fluid requirements secondary to differences in BSA to weight ratio and require larger volumes of urine for excretion of waste products. The volume required in the first 24 hours for the burned pediatric patient is estimated using the Galveston Formula (established at the Shriners Institute for Burned Children, Galveston, TX):

$$[2000 \text{ cc times TBSA}] + [5000 \text{ cc times burn surface area } (\text{m}^2)]$$

$$\text{where TBSA } (\text{m}^2) = 0.007184 \times (\text{height in cm})^{0.725} \times (\text{weight in kg})^{0.425}$$

$$\text{BSA } (\text{m}^2) = \text{TBSA} \times \%\ \text{surface area burned (i.e., rule of nines)}$$

The rate of infusion for Parkland and Galveston formula:

- Half of the determined volume is given within the first 8 hours of the time of the burn.
- The remaining volume is given during the succeeding 16 hours.

Fluid requirements beyond the first 24 hours are determined based on the patient's weight and evaporative losses, and adjusted according to the patient's response (i.e., urine output). Maintenance volume of fluid is calculated in L/day as

- 100 mL/kg for first 10 kg
- 50 mL/kg for second 10 kg
- 20 mL/kg for each additional kg of body weight

In addition:

Evaporated losses related to the burn wounds/per day

$$= 3750 \text{ mL} \times \text{BSA}^{*} (\text{m}^2)$$

* (BSA burn surface area)

This volume is then added to the maintenance volume and divided over 24 hours.

Alternatively, the maintenance volume per day in the postacute resuscitation period is calculated:

$$[1500 \text{ mL} \times \text{TBSA}^{*} (\text{m}^2)] + [3750 \text{ mL} \times \text{BSA} (\text{m}^2)]$$

*(TBSA total body surface area)

Ultimately, this calculation should be adjusted to ensure adequate end-organ perfusion as monitored by the patient's urine output, which should be >0.5 cc/kg/h for adults or 1 cc/kg/h for children.

Burn Patient Triage

The spectrum in severity of burn injury varies from mild to fatal. Triage of the burn patient includes outpatient management, inpatient management, management by a trauma service, or referral to a specialized burn center. The criteria for referral to a burn center are outlined in **Table 5–3**.

The criteria for the management of burn victims as outpatients include the following:

- Burns are $<10\%$ partial thickness burns without inhalation injury.
- Patients are responsive to oral analgesics.

Table 5–3 Burn Unit Referral Criteria

• Partial thickness burns >10% TBSA • Burns involving the face, hands, feet, genitalia, perineum, or major joints • Third-degree burns of any age group • Electrical burns, including lightning injury • Chemical burns • Inhalation injury • Burns in patients with preexisting medical disorders that could complicate management, prolong recovery, or affect outcome • Any patient with burns and associated trauma in which the burn injury poses the greater immediate risk of morbidity and mortality • Burned children in hospitals without qualified personnel or equipment for children • Burn injury in patients who will require special social, emotional, or long-term rehabilitative intervention

Source: From Committee on Trauma, Resources for Optimal Care of the Injured Patient. Chicago: American College of Surgeons; 2006. Reprinted with permission.

- Victims are compliant patients, who will care for their wounds and present for follow-up evaluation within 3 to 5 days.
- There is no immediate or delayed risk to specialized areas (i.e., circumferential burns).

All other burn victims require hospital admission for more extensive treatment or monitoring. At times, patients with minor burns must be admitted for pain control or personal safety/caution, as in the case of abuse or patients with multiple preexisting comorbidities or trauma.

Burn Wound Management

The patient should be premedicated with analgesics prior to wound treatment to decrease discomfort and increase patient cooperation.

General Principles

- Cleanse wound of particles and débride devitalized tissue
- Initiate tetanus prophylaxis
- Daily or twice-daily wound cleansing and dressing
- Antibiotics only for gross soft tissue infection
- Aggressive pain control

Use chlorhexidine, 0.5% silver nitrate combined with chlorhexidine gluconate, normal saline, or soap and water to cleanse the burn wound. To prevent wound infection and deeper wound conversion, topical antimicrobials are used until epithelization of the wound is complete. The topical antimicrobials are provided via gauze applications, ointments, creams, or solutions; dressings are changed at least twice a day. Commonly used topical antimicrobials are outlined in **Table 5–4** and antimicrobial dressings in **Table 5–5**.

Outpatient Wound Dressings

Epidermal, First-Degree Burns

- Heal spontaneously with little intervention required
- Moisturize the wound to alleviate pain

Partial-Thickness Burns, Superficial Second-Degree Burns

- Treat blisters
  - Minor blisters over a small surface require no intervention
  - Large, tense, turbid, painful blisters
    - Using aseptic technique, aspirate with a large bore needle, leaving epidermis as a biologic dressing
    - Débride epidermis if wounds are contaminated
    - Clean wound thoroughly and dress using
      - Gauze
      - Xeroform gauze
      - Biobrane (UDL Laboratories, Inc., Rockford, IL) – for clean scald burns
- Apply soft bulky gauze dressing
- Administer analgesic
- Follow up in 2 to 3 days. If the patient is free of pain and wounds are healing, then instruct the patient or caregiver on how to continue dressing changes at home.

Mid to Deep Dermal Burns, Second- and Third-Degree Burns

- Clean wound thoroughly with chlorhexidine
- Débride superficial devitalized tissue
- Dress wounds with antimicrobial material

Table 5–4 Characteristics of Commonly Used Topical Antimicrobial Ointments

Antimicrobial Agent	Usage and Characteristics	Available Forms	Antimicrobial Coverage	Local Effects	Systemic Effects
Silver sulfadiazine	Mid-dermal burns Deep burns Does not penetrate eschar	Cream solution	*S. aureus* *E. coli* *Klebsiella* *Pseudomonas aeruginosa* *Proteus* *Candida albicans*	Painless application Cooling effect Harmless yellow-gray "pseudo eschar"	Recoverable leukopenia
Mafenide acetate	Deep burns Burn with invasive infection Penetrates burn eschar	Cream solution	Activity against most gram-positive species *Clostridia* MRSA minimal antifungal activity	Painful maculopapular rash in 5% of patients	Hyperchloremic Metabolic acidosis Carbonic anhydrase inhibitor Moderate to severe compensatory hyperventilation
Silver nitrate	Mid-dermal to deep burns	Cream solution	Efficacy is similar to silver sulfadiazine *Staphylococcus* *Pseudomonas* Gram-negative aerobes	Painless Causes black staining reaction with contact Clean wound and reapply q2h to prevent histotoxicity	Hyponatremia Hypokalemia Methemoglobinemia

Table 5–4 (*Continued*)

Antimicrobial Agent	Usage and Characteristics	Available Forms	Antimicrobial Coverage	Local Effects	Systemic Effects
Mupirocin (Bactroban*)	Superficial burns Facial burns Hand burns	Cream	*Staphylococcus* *Streptococcus* Enteric *Pseudomonas* MRSA	Increases wound healing half-life by 2 d	
Bacitracin/ polymyxin	Superficial burns facial burns hand burns well tolerated	Cream	Decreases S. *aureus* colonization	Local irritation to local tissues after 72 h of use	
Gentamycin sulfate	Ear burns with exposed cartilage	0.1% Water-soluble cream	Gram-negative Enteric *Pseudomonas*		

*GlaxoSmithKline, Mississauga, Ontario, Canada.

Table 5–5 Antimicrobial Dressings

Antimicrobial Dressing	Characteristics	Uses	Coverage	Notes on Usage
Biobrane	Silicone, nylon, collagen matrix Impermeable to bacteria Controls evaporative water loss Permeable to topical antibiotics	Clean superficial burns (scald)	None	Membrane may trap infection Close monitoring warranted Can be combined with antimicrobial ointments
XeroForm	3% Bismuth tribromophenate in petrolatum blend on fine mesh gauze Non-adherent Conforms to body contours Deodorizing agent	Superficial burns Hand burns	Bacteriostatic	Can be combined with antimicrobial ointments
Acticoat*	Thin sheet of flexible rayon/polyester bonded to polyethylene mesh Coated with nanocrystalline silver film Silver ions released and sustains antimicrobial effect for 24–48 h Painless No systemic toxicity	Mid- to deep-dermal burns	Spectrum is similar to silver nitrate *Staphylococcus* *Pseudomonas* Gram-negative aerobes	Black discoloration with contact Change every 48 h

*Smith & Nephew plc, London, England.

- Silvadene (Sanofi-Aventis Pharmaceuticals, Paris, France)
    - Sulfamylon (Mylan Laboratories, Canonsburg, PA) – for burns with eschar formation
- Apply soft bulky gauze dressing
- Administer analgesic
- Administer antibiotic (Bactrim [Roche Pharmaceuticals, Nutley, NJ] DS PO b.i.d.) for signs of infection (i.e., cellulitis)
- Follow up in 3 to 5 days
- Refer for possible excision and grafting

Management of Burns to Specific Anatomic Regions

Hand Burns

- Assess for neurovascular compromise
- Perform escharotomies on deep injury
- Stabilization of open joint deformities with K-wires
- Elevate
- Splint in position of safety
- Refer patient for occupational therapy
- Wound care
    - Apply Xeroform gauze
    - Use Biobrane glove for superficial burns
- Full-thickness burns are referred for early excision and grafting to prevent scarring and contracture leading to dysfunction.

Facial Burns

- Evaluate for inhalation injury
- Assess for injury to eyes and ears
- Keep head elevated
- For superficial and deep burns:
    - Daily cleansing
    - Apply bacitracin ointment
- For full-thickness burns:
    - Allow 5 to 7 days of healing before committing to grafting
    - Cover temporarily with amnion or bacitracin

Ear Burns

- Assess external canal and drum for otitis media or externa and tympanic membrane perforation

- Apply topical sulfamylon or Gentamycin (A.G. Scientific, San Diego, CA) ointment to exposed cartilage
  - Beware of chondritis
  - Avoid placing pillows under the head

Eyelid Burns

- Irrigate with buffered saline solution
- Perform fluorescein examination to identify corneal injury; consult an ophthalmologist
- Superficial burns
  - Thin layer of bacitracin ointment – do not contaminate eye
- Full-thickness burns
  - Excise and graft with full thickness skin early to prevent ectropion and corneal exposure

Burns to the Genitalia

- Insert Foley catheter to maintain patency of urethra
- Penile escharotomy for circumferential injury
- Partial-thickness burns heal spontaneously with conservative management – amnion, Polysporin (Pfizer Pharmaceuticals, New York, NY), bacitracin
- Refer full-thickness burns for grafting, dress with Silvadene (Sanofi-Aventis Pharmaceuticals, Paris, France)

Escharotomy

Late tissue edema may lead to vascular compromise secondary to decreased elasticity of a burn scar. This is particularly hazardous in deep burns of the extremities and circumferential burns of the chest wall. An escharotomy is performed early for circumferential deep dermal and full-thickness burns to the extremities and chest. Generally, escharotomies should be performed by a physician experienced in the procedure to decrease morbidity.

Procedure (Fig. 5–8)

- Use electrocautery or a scalpel to incise the burned skin
- Extend down through eschar into the subcutaneous fat
- Cut mid-medially or mid-laterally

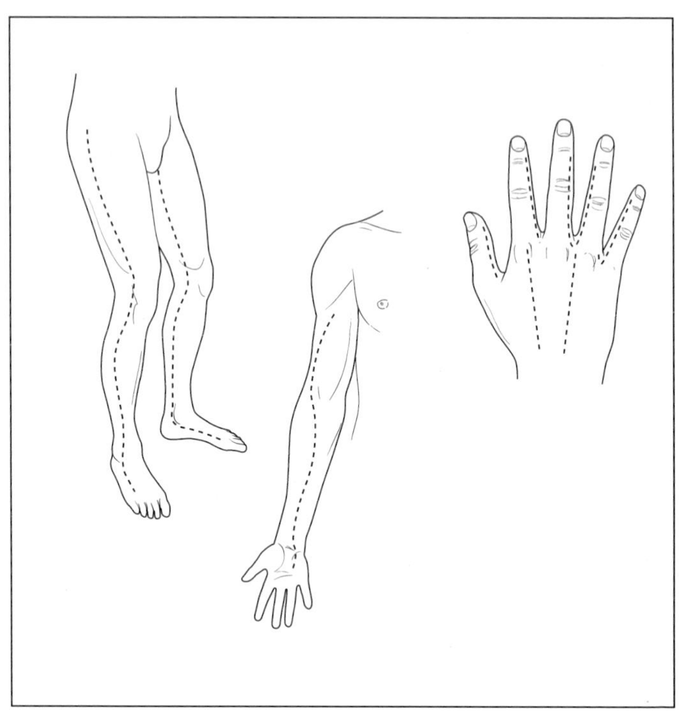

Figure 5–8 Incision locations for escharotomy.

- Extend the incision the length of constricting burn eschar and across involved joints
- Avoid major vessels, nerves, tendons, and pressure surfaces

Associated Conditions

Inhalation Injury

The leading cause of death in fires is smoke inhalation, not burns. Inhalation injury is present in one third of burn patients and doubles the mortality rate from burns.

Signs and Symptoms of Inhalation Injury

- Anatomic distortion of the face and neck edema
- Inability of the patient to clear secretions
- Altered mental status

- Decreased oxygenation
- Increased carboxyhemoglobin
- Lactic acidosis

Management of Inhalation Injury

- Evaluate patient for intubation
- Perform a fiberoptic laryngoscopy and bronchoscopy for diagnosis and soot/secretion removal
- 100% oxygen supplementation
- Assess for carbon monoxide poisoning
- Elevate chest/head to 20 to 30 degrees at all times
- Liberal use of bronchodilators such as albuterol
- Transfer patient to a burn center or critical care setting

For advanced management of severely burned airway:

  - Intubate; apply positive pressure ventilation
  - Positive end expiratory pressure (PEEP); maintain patency of smaller airways
  - Give the patient *N*-acetyl cysteine
  - Administer nebulized heparin
  - Transfer patient to a burn center or critical care setting

Carbon Monoxide Toxicity

Carbon monoxide toxicity is one of the leading causes of death associated with fires and is produced in the process of O_2 combustion. Carbon monoxide preferentially binds to hemoglobin in place of oxygen and forms carboxyhemoglobin (COHb), which shifts the oxyhemoglobin dissociation curve to the left, reducing oxygen delivery. Signs and symptoms of carbon monoxide poisoning are outlined in **Table 5–6**.

Management of Carbon Monoxide Toxicity

- Administer high-flow oxygen by mask (FiO_2 100%) until carboxyhemoglobin is $<10\%$
- For obtunded patients:
  - Intubate
  - 90 to 100% oxygen via positive pressure ventilation

Table 5–6 Symptoms of Carbon Monoxide Poisoning

COHb (%)	Symptoms
0–5	Normal value
15–20	Headache, confusion
20–40	Disorientation, fatigue, nausea, visual changes
40–60	Hallucination, combativeness, coma, shock state
>60	Mortality >50%

If the patient is not responding to 100% oxygen:

- Consider advanced modes of ventilating
  - Volume diffusive respirator (VDR; Percussionaire, Sandpoint, ID)
  - Bilevel IVR ventilation
    - Hyperbaric therapy

Types of Burns

Electrical Burns

Electrical burn injury results from a spectrum of low- to high-voltage electrical exposure from lightning, direct electrical contact (electrocutions), and electrical arching. The passage of the electric current through the body causes thermoelectric burns. Flash burns are thermal burns caused by the heat generated by an arc of electricity. Flame burns may result from ignition of clothing. Moreover, the systemic manifestations of electrical injury are generally greater than the local tissue injury and are potentially fatal. The systemic complications of electrical injury are outlined in **Table 5–7**.

Management of Electrical Burns

- Acute airway management and resuscitation
- Admit for observation or refer to burn unit
- 24-Hour continuous cardiac monitoring and serial assessment of myocardial enzyme leak (creatine kinase [CK], troponin, lactate dehydrogenase [LDH])
- Evaluation for rhabdomyolysis and myoglobinuria
  - Diagnosis
    - Increased urine pigment – red

Table 5–7 Systemic Effects of Electrical Exposure

Cardiovascular
Changes in the permeability of myocyte membranes
Cardiac arrest and ventricular fibrillation
Conduction defects
Creation of arrhythmogenic foci due to myocardial necrosis
Neurological
Loss of consciousness
Confusion
Amnesia
Seizures
Visual disturbances
Delayed onset paralysis
Respiratory
Apnea from damage to cerebral respiratory center
Renal
Acute tubular necrosis
Myoglobinuria
Musculoskeletal
Myonecrosis
Rhabdomyolysis
Compartment syndrome
Fractures and dislocations from tetany

        - Urine dipstick is heme positive, but no RBCs are seen on microscopic evaluation
        - Increased urine myoglobin
    - Treatment
        - Increase renal perfusion
        - Aggressive resuscitation
            - To maintain adequate urinary output, at least 0.5 cc/kg/h of urine (35 cc/h for a 70-kg patient), but preferably 50 to 100 cc/h
            - Mannitol 0.25 to 1 g/kg over 20 minutes q4 to 6h
        - Alkalinize urine
            - Add sodium bicarbonate – 1 to 2 mEq/kg/d to IV fluids; adjust dose according to serum and urinary pH
- Evaluation of the limbs for compartment syndrome and need for escharotomy

- MRI or CT evaluation for deeper injuries
- Ophthalmologic and otoscopic evaluation
- CT scan of the head is indicated in all high-voltage injuries
- Thorough evaluation for hidden injury; spinal cord injury; blunt thoracic, abdominal trauma
- Supportive care

Chemical Burns

Approximately 3% of all burns are secondary to chemical exposure, and 30% of burn deaths are due to chemical injuries. More than 25,000 home or industrial products are available that can cause chemical injury. The resultant injury from chemical solutions causes tissue protein coagulation and necrosis. The offending agent continues to destroy the tissues until the agent is neutralized or completely removed. Deeper penetration of the chemical compound can result in severe systemic toxicity. Common household agents and neutralizing substances are outlined in **Table 5–8**.

Table 5–8 Common Household Agents Associated with Chemical Injury

Agent	Common Use	Treatment
Phenol	Deodorant Sanitizer Plastics Dyes Fertilizers Explosives Disinfectants	Polyethylene glycol Vegetable oil Bacitracin ointment
Phosphorous	Explosives (fireworks) Poisons Insecticides Fertilizers	Lavage with 1% copper sulfate Castor Oil
Sodium hypochlorite	Bleach	Milk
Potassium permanganate	Deodorizer Disinfectant	Egg white Paste Starch
Lye	Drain cleaner	Water lavage Mafenide acetate
Chromic acid	Metal cleansing	Water lavage

Characteristics of Chemical Burns

- Acid burns
  - Tissue damage leads to coagulation necrosis.
  - Cause exothermic reactions with exposure
  - Associated with hypocalcemia and hypomagnesemia
  - Exposure may lead to inhalational injury.
  - Systemic toxicity may lead to hepatic or renal failure.
- Alkali burns
  - Constituent of lye exposure
  - Tissue damage leads to liquefaction necrosis and saponification of fats.
  - Tissue injury appears less severe than the actual depth of injury.
  - Alkali burns are associated with a higher incidence of systemic toxicity.

Management of Chemical Burns

- Obtain a thorough history to identify offending agent
- Carefully inspect hands, face, and eyes
- Remove all clothing and sources of chemical contact
- Immediately irrigate with water (except phenol). If the patient presents with a severe chemical exposure, plan on irrigation for hours in a shower (especially lye exposures). Small exposures can be treated with smaller volumes of fluid. Always err on the side of more fluid irrigation than needed.
- Resuscitate based on amount of surface exposed and monitor urine output
- Consider antidote – refer to toxicologist, poison control center, or local burn center for assistance with management
- Monitor electrolytes and obtain blood gas to assess for systemic toxicity
- Provide supportive therapy in a monitored environment for large burns
- Once irrigated, dress wounds with Silvadene
- Refer patients to burn centers and specialized facilities for excision and graft of mid-dermal to full-thickness chemical burns

Treatments for Specific Chemical Burns

- Sodium or lithium metal, mustard gas
  - Cover with oil, sand, or class D fire extinguisher; excise immediately
  - Do not irrigate with water
- Phenol
  - Wipe with polyethylene glycol
  - Do not irrigate with water
- Phosphorous
  - Copper sulfate irrigation
- Hydrofluoric acid
  - Irrigate with 5% calcium gluconate or massage with 2.5% calcium gluconate gel. If pain persists, inject 5% calcium gluconate subcutaneously until pain is relieved.
  - Magnesium sulfate subcutaneous injection may also be used.

Chemical Burn Triage

Due to the unique mechanism of chemical burn injury, specialty assistance should be sought from the Poison Control Center (telephone 800-222-1222) or a local burn unit. Patients with the following characteristics should be admitted and possibly referred to a burn unit (**Table 5–3**):

- Chemical injury >15% TBSA
- Full-thickness burns
- Burns to the perineum, eye, foot, hand
- Multiple comorbidities
- Patients at extremes of age

♦ Frostbite

Cold injury results from both tissue freezing (frostbite) and nonfreezing injury (trench foot). Frostbite is the result of tissue freezing after exposure to temperatures <28°F (−2°C). At such temperatures, ice crystals form intracellularly that cause tissue destruction and intravascular crystals contribute to microvascular occlusion. The pathogenesis of trench foot is secondary to exposure, usually of an extremity to a moist environment at temperatures 32 to 50°F (1 to

10°C) for long periods. This creates a scenario of excessive heat loss in the involved region. There is also ischemic perfusion secondary to vasoconstriction. Patients with cold thermal injury will commonly experience severe pain, pruritus, numbness, paresthesias, and hyperemia, which may last up to 6 weeks.

Management of Cold Thermal Injury

- Rapid rewarming of the involved area
  - Water immersion – heated to 104°F (40°C)
- Administer
  - Parenteral analgesics
  - Tetanus prophylaxis
  - Systemic prostaglandin inhibitors – ibuprofen
  - Topical thromboxane inhibitors, e.g., aloe vera
- Débride necrotic tissue
  - Whirlpool (hydrotherapy débridement)
  - Allow complete wound demarcation before committing to radical surgical débridement
- Elevate affected areas
- Begin early passive range of motion to all involved extremities
- Dress wound twice a day and protect from further injury

6

The Traumatized Face

No matter how severe or traumatic the facial injury (**Fig. 6–1**), these patients still require an appropriate trauma evaluation beginning with the ABCs (airway, breathing, circulation). Facial injuries are rarely life threatening; the patient must be evaluated for all other serious injuries before attempting repair. Usually treatment of any intraabdominal, thoracic, or neurologic injury takes precedence. Coordinate care between the trauma, thoracic, vascular, ENT, orthopedic, ophthalmic, and neurosurgical services.

Any exam should start with a detailed medical, surgical, social, and previous craniofacial injury history. The mechanism of injury should be ascertained to gauge the force of contact and determine where potential fractures or soft tissue injuries may be. Other considerations include loss of consciousness, breathing difficulties, and hearing trouble.

♦ Airway Establishment

Avoid nasal intubation in patients suspected of having a skull base fracture or excessive midface trauma. Elective oral endotracheal intubation should be considered in patients with severe pan-facial trauma, especially in the midface and mandible. Patients with large posterior base of tongue injuries should also be electively intubated. Any intubation should be done with due consideration of the cervical spine (C-spine): 10% of facial traumas harbor a C-spine injury. Tracheogtomy should be considered in complex cases, particularly when nasal or oral trauma preclude upper airway connulations.

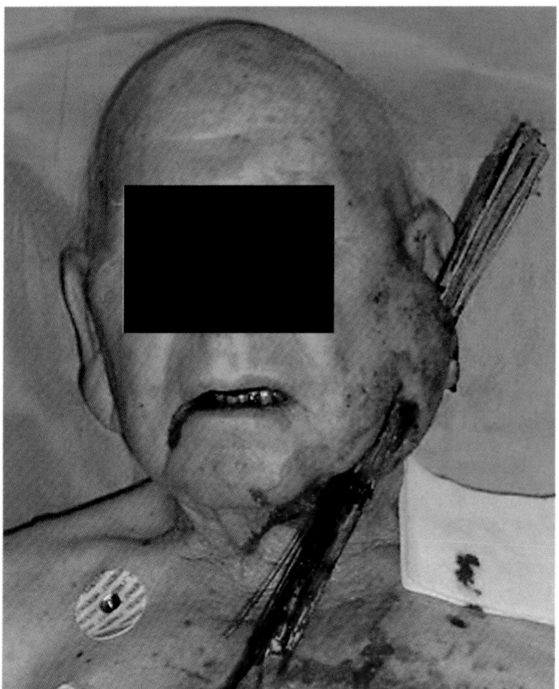

Figure 6–1 Patient impaled with a stick.

♦ Patient Evaluation

Examination

Remove all necessary articles of clothing and jewelry. Irrigate all dirt, foreign bodies, and dry crusted blood to avoid obscurity of the injury. Note all lacerations, asymmetries, bleeding, bruising, or foreign bodies. An organized systematic approach is recommended to avoid any missed injuries. Check for

- raccoon eyes (periorbital ecchymosis) – skull base fracture
- battle sign (postauricular ecchymosis) – skull base fracture
- otorrhea – skull base fracture, condylar fracture
- hemotympanum – skull base fracture
- perforated tympanic membrane

- epistaxis – nasal fracture
- CSF rhinorrhea – cribriform plate fracture, NOE fracture
- intraoral
  - edema
  - bleeding
  - gingival bleeding
  - fractured/loose/displaced teeth
  - dental caries
    - septal hematoma

Nasal Palpation

- Tenderness
- Crepitus/subcutaneous emphysema
- Bony step-offs
  - Scalp – gently palpate to uncover depressions/crepitus
  - Forehead – frontal sinus fracture
  - Orbital rim
  - NOE (naso-orbito ethmoid) – palpate intranasally and inward from medial canthus-bony movement to diagnose NOE fracture
  - Nasal bridge
  - Zygoma
  - Maxilla – gently depress the maxilla with both thumbs to rule out Le Fort fractures. If mobile, grab the central incisors between thumb and index finger with one hand and hold the nasal spine with other hand. Movement of the entire dental alveolus indicates a Le Fort I fracture; movement of the nasal bridge indicates Le Fort II or III.
  - Mandible – preauricular pain on palpation can be indicative of a condylar fracture
  - Neck exam – performed with caution in relation to the C-spine

Ophthalmic Assessment

- Inspection
  - Corrective lens (contacts or eyeglasses)
  - Enophthalmos/exophthalmos

- Retrobulbar hematoma
- Interpupillary distance – normally 30 to 32 mm
- Hyphema - blood layering in the inferior aspect of the anterior chamber. An ophthalmologist should be consulted immediately based upon the potential increase in intraocular pressure.
- Cornea abrasion
- Subconjunctival hemorrhage
- Chemosis – scleral edema
- Upper eyelid ptosis
- Fat protrusion

- Visual acuity
  - Test each eye separately by measuring patient's ability to read legible fine print (ID card)
    - Diplopia
    - Red color saturation – *first color affected* in impending optic nerve injury
    - Compare and contrast red color perception in each eye individually
  - Variation in exam may indicate optic nerve injury
- Extraocular muscle function – muscle entrapment: forced duction test (Chapter 9)
- Pupillary response – reactivity, dilated, constricted
  - Consensual light response
    - If light is exposed to one eye, there should be ipsilateral and contralateral constriction of the pupils.
    - An injured eye may be fixed and dilated secondary to intrinsic damage to that eye, but maintain normal afferent optic nerve function. In this scenario, there will be loss of ipsilateral pupillary constriction; however, contralateral constriction is maintained.
  - When contralateral papillary constriction is lost, this indicates an afferent pupillary defect in the affected eye.
    - In a patient suspected of an afferent pupillary defect, exposing the unaffected eye to light will cause both pupils to constrict.
    - When the light is brought back to the affected pupil, this pupil will dilate (due to consensual relaxation), instead of constricting, confirming an afferent pupillary defect in this eye.

- Medial/lateral canthal tendon stability: traction test – pull laterally on medial aspect of lower eyelid; laxity is indicative of medial canthal tendon disruption

Immediate attention should be paid to any signs of acute optic compressive neuropathy, penetrating globe injuries, or vision loss. Any questionable injury or condition warrants an ophthalmologic consult/evaluation.

Motor/Sensory Assessment

After soft tissue and bony assessment is complete, test for motor and sensory deficits (**Table 6–1**). Assess the patient's occlusion and have the patient compare this with their preinjury occlusion. Abnormal occlusion is highly suggestive of mandibular, maxillary, and Le Fort fractures. Test all muscles of facial expression and follow with a detailed sensory exam.

- Motor
  - Temporal
  - Zygomatic
  - Buccal
  - Marginal mandibular
  - Cervical
- Sensory—Trigenical
  - V_1
    - Supraorbital nerve
    - Supratrochlear nerve
    - Lacrimal nerve
    - Infratrochlear nerve
    - External nasal branch of anterior ethmoidal nerve
  - V_2
    - Infraorbital nerve
    - Zygomaticofacial nerve
    - Zygomatic temporal nerve
  - V_3
    - Mental nerve
    - Buccal nerve
    - Auriculotemporal nerve

Table 6–1 Evaluation of Cranial Nerve Function in Patients with Facial Trauma

CN	Name	Innervation	Functional Test	Dysfunction	Potential Injuries
I	Olfactory	Smell	Coffee, perfume, alcohol	Lack of smell	Cribriform plate of the ethmoid bone
II	Optic	Sight	Visual acuity	Blindness, nonreactive pupil	Orbital apex syndrome, posterior orbital vault fracture, edema, hematoma
III	Oculomotor	Papillary constrictors, levator palpebrae superioris; the superior, inferior, and medial recti; inferior oblique muscles	Ocular movement, papillary constriction	Ptosis, outward turned eye (exotropia), diplopia, blurred vision, nonreactive pupil	Posterior orbital vault fracture involving SOF
IV	Trochlear	Superior oblique	Allows viewing tip of nose	Exotropia without ptosis, diplopia with walking down stairs, blurred vision	Posterior orbital vault fracture involving SOF

(Continued)

Table 6–1 *(Continued)*

CN	Name	Innervation	Functional Test	Dysfunction	Potential Injuries
V	Trigeminal V_1 – Ophthalmic	Sensory to forehead	Forehead sensation	Anesthesia	Posterior orbital vault fracture involving SOF
	Trigeminal V_2 – Maxillary	Sensation to midface	Cheek sensation	Anesthesia	Fractures of the maxilla
	Trigeminal V_3 – Mandibular	Sensation to lower teeth, cheek, and chin; motor to muscles of mastication	Sensation over lower third of face, bite	Anesthesia of the lower third of face, weak bite	Fractures of the mandible
VI	Abducens	Motor to lateral rectus	Abduct eye	Inward turned eye (esotropia), diplopia, blurred vision	Posterior orbital vault fracture involving SOF
VII	Facial, temporal, zygomatic, buccal, mandibular, cervical	Motor to facial muscles, taste to anterior two-thirds of tongue	Facial expression – raise eyebrows, close eyes, smile, puff out cheeks	Total facial paralysis or selective depending on branch	Lacerations or avulsions to main nerve (near styloid mastoid foramen) or associated branches

Table 6–1 *(Continued)*

CN	Name	Innervation	Functional Test	Dysfunction	Potential InjuriesIV
VIII	Vestibulo-cochlear	Hearing/vestibular functions	Hearing	Hearing loss even with tuning fork on mastoid	Rule out CN injury vs. external or middle ear injury
	Glossophar-yngeal	Sensory innervation of the posterior third of the tongue and the pharynx	Gag reflex	Loss of sensation to posterior third of the tongue and the pharynx	
X	Vagus	Visceral, sensory, motor and parasympathetic innervations	Gag reflex, swallowing, hoarseness with recurrent laryngeal nerve injury	Loss of gag reflex, uvula deviation to noninjured side	
XI	Accessory	Motor innervation to SCM and trapezius	Shrug shoulders, lateral resistance to face	Weak ipsilateral shoulder shrug, weak ipsilateral SCM function	Deep lateral neck lacerations
XII	Hypoglossal	Motor innervation to the tongue	Tongue protrusion	Deviation of the tongue to injured side	Deep submental lacerations

Abbreviations: CN, central nerve; SCM, sternocleidomastoid; SOF super orbital fissure,.

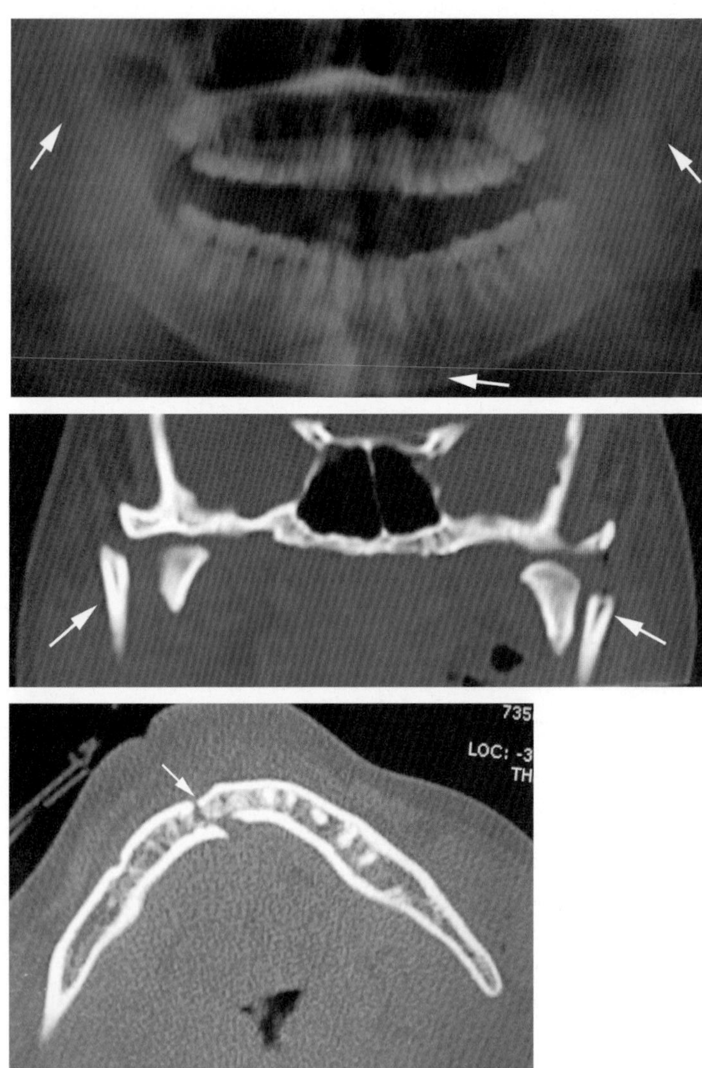

Figure 6–2 (A) Panorex radiograph of a mandible fractur. Arrows point to bilateral condyle fractures and parasymphyseal fracture. **(B)** CT scan of fracture demonstrating the bilateral condyle fracture. **(C)** CT scan demonstrating parasymphyseal fracture

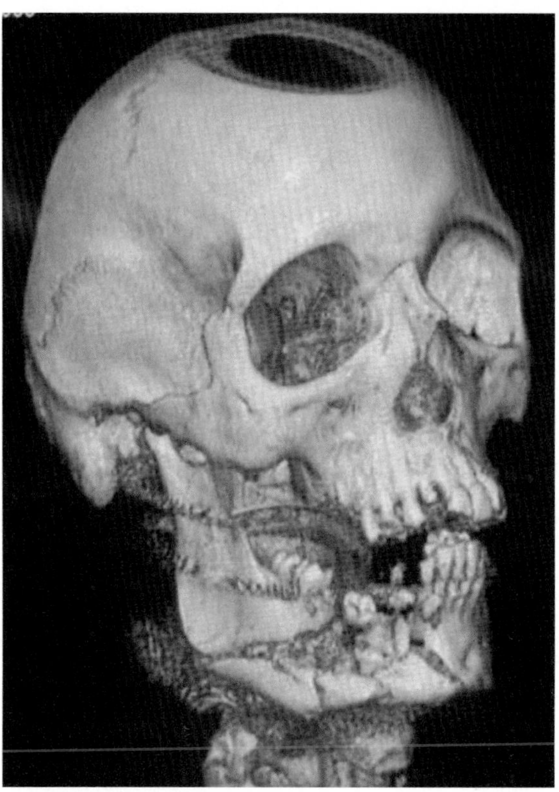

Figure 6–3 3D reconstruction of the facial bones.

Radiographic Evaluation

If facial fractures are suspected, a CT scan of the face is warranted, especially if the patient is to be scanned for other potential injuries (**Fig. 6–2**). High-resolution (axial and coronal) views should be obtained through the orbits and 3D reconstructions obtained if possible (**Fig. 6–3**).

In case of a possible mandible fracture, Panorex radiograph is the only plain film that should still be routinely obtained even if a CT scan of the face is also obtained (**Fig. 6–2**). Panorex radiograph films are excellent for evaluating fractures, condyles, and provide a single plain film view of the entire mandible. They are also useful in evaluating dentition such as impacted molars. Panorex films are poor for evaluating symphyseal fractures.

Additional plain films (rarely used) include

- *Waters view* PA view that requires neck extension. Occipital-mental projection that optimizes superior and inferior orbital rims, nasal bones, zygoma, and maxillary sinuses
- *Caldwell view* PA view that requires neck flexion. Occipital-orbital projection that optimizes frontal bones and sinus, lateral walls of the maxillary sinus, orbital rims, and zygomaticofrontal sutures
- *Lateral view* optimizes anterior frontal sinus wall, anterior and posterior maxillary sinus walls
- *Submental view* optimizes view of zygomatic arches

♦ Acute Management

Wound and Hemorrhage Control

Large deep lacerations can first be treated with irrigation followed by application of pressure to control bleeding. Active arterial bleeders can be tied off or suture ligated with 4–0 Vicryl (Ethicon, Somerville, NJ) suture. Wounds can be extended with a scalpel to gain exposure. Because of the extensive collateral vascular supply of the face and scalp, even lacerations to the facial artery can be ligated if necessary to control bleeding. To avoid injury to nerves and other vital structures, do not blindly clamp any vessels. If direct visualization is not possible due to excessive bleeding, place 4 × 4 gauze on the wound, place pressure on the wound, and take the patient to the operating room.

Epistaxis can be controlled with anteroposterior nasal packing. Obtain a nasal speculum and bayonet forceps along with Cottonoid (Codman & Shurtleff, Raynham, MA) soaked in epinephrine (1:200,000) (**Fig. 6–4A**). Four percent cocaine may also be used, but with great caution. If Cottonoid is not available, cut Xeroform gauze into strips and layer them into the nasal cavity. Under direct visualization using a nasal speculum, layer (do not stuff or pack) the gauze or Cottonoid into the posterior nasal pharynx (**Fig. 6–4**). When nasal packing is used, start the patient on prophylactic antibiotics to prevent streptococcal toxic shock syndrome.

Occasionally, midface and mandibular fractures can result in severe bleeding. Common vascular structures include the maxillary artery, alveolar artery, retromandibular vein, facial artery/vein or buccal branches of the facial artery. Access to these structures is difficult

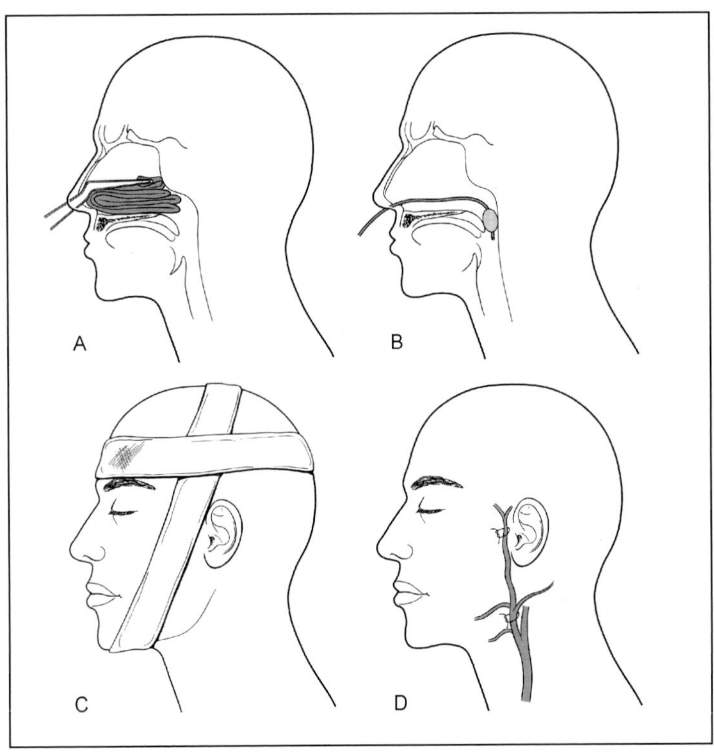

Figure 6–4 Techniques for achieving hemostasis. **(A)** Anterior nasal packing. **(B)** Posterior nasal packing. **(C)** Barton bandage head wrap. **(D)** Selective arterial ligation or embolization.

and attempts should be made to obtain some crude reduction to tamponade the bleeding. A Barton bandage can be applied using Kerlix (Kendall Co., Mansfield, MA) reinforced with an Ace bandage to apply compression to the face. The Kerlix is wrapped coronally multiple times to hold the mandible in occlusion, then wrapped around the forehead. Reinforce with an Ace wrap (**Fig. 6–4C**).

A Bridle wire (25-gauge wire passed around two teeth flanking a fracture) can be used to help stabilize a fracture. Stabilization will also help to offset the patient's pain. A more effective technique may be Essig wiring. This involves passing a 25-gauge wire around two teeth on either side of the fracture and then placing interdental wires above and below the first wire.

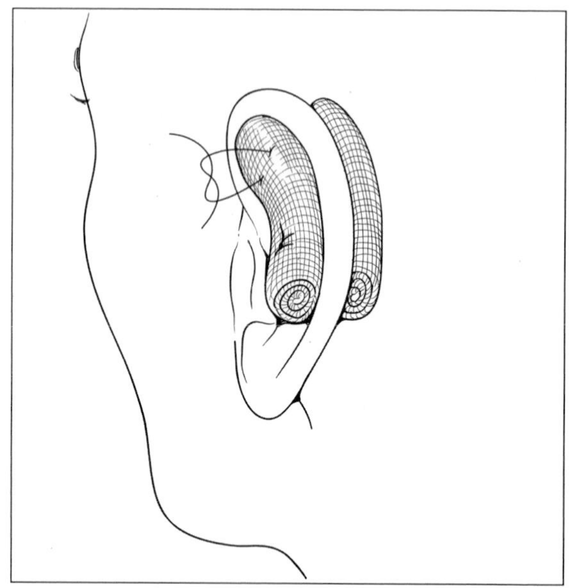

Figure 6–5 Ear bolster dressing technique.

Nasal septal hematomas need to be drained in the emergency room to prevent septal necrosis. Using an 18-gauge needle or 11-blade scalpel, make a small perforation in the mucosa with a nasal speculum under direct visualization. Evacuate the hematoma and apply a compressive dressing (Xeroform layered packing with bacitracin ointment) to prevent reaccumulation (**Fig. 6–4A**). Note that if there was no epistasis at the time of the injury, the presence of a nasal bone fracture is less likely.

Auricular hematomas should be treated like septal hematomas. Drain with a scalpel or an 18-gauge needle (aspirate) and apply pressure dressing. Bolster the ear with rolled up Xeroform gauze sutured in place with through and through 2–0/3–0 nylon or Prolene (Ethicon, Somerville, NJ) (**Fig. 6–5**).

Acute optic compressive neuropathy requires emergent lateral canthotomy (**Fig. 6–6**) along with mannitol, acetazolamide, and methylprednisolone to decrease intraocular pressure and to control orbital nerve edema.

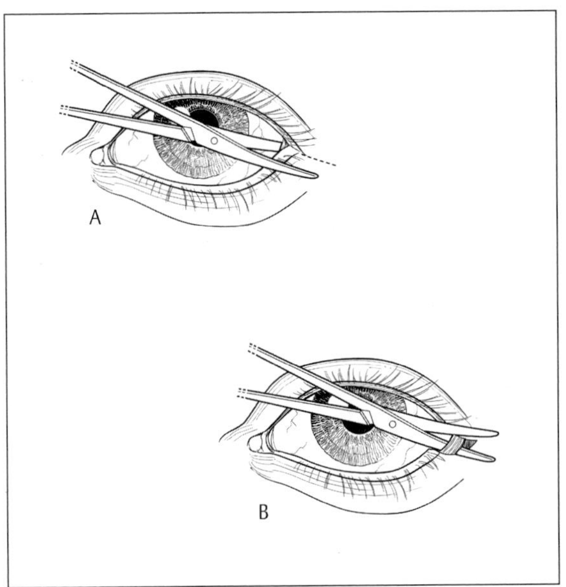

Figure 6–6 (A) Lateral canthotomy. **(B)** Release of the lateral canthal tendon.

- Mannitol: 50 to 100 g (1.5 gm/kg) of 5% solution IV over 2 hours repeat dose to maintain urine output (>30 to 50 cc/hour) with a maximum of 200 gm/day. Test dose with 200 mg/kg.
- Acetazolamide: 250 mg PO qAM or 5 mg/kg IV q24h
- Methylprednisolone: Loading dose = 30 mg/kg, then in 2 hours 15 mg/kg q6h

Treatment Sequence and Timing

Polytrauma patients will be admitted to the trauma service. Bony repair is delayed until the patient is stable. If possible, repair should be performed immediately to avoid excessive edema or delayed from 10 days to 2 weeks after injury to allow the edema to subside. Soft tissue injuries should be irrigated and repaired within 8 hours. Do not leave open wounds on the face to granulate; attempt closure by any means. Remember that closure does not need to be definitive because revisions can be made later during bony repair.

7

Facial Lacerations

Facial soft tissue injuries constitute approximately 3 million visits to emergency departments in the United States each year. Motor vehicle accidents (MVAs) have historically comprised the majority of these injuries. With state and federal seat belt laws, the incidence of MVA-related injuries has recently decreased. However, the overall incidence of facial injuries has remained constant due to sports and job-related injuries, animal bites, and domestic- and interpersonal-violence-related factors.

♦ Assessment

The immediate priority for patients with facial injuries is to control the airway and any bleeding. Detailed evaluation of the facial trauma patient is outlined in Chapters 6 and 10.

The physical examination proceeds with inspection and palpation of the patient. Using a systematic approach from the scalp to the base of the clavicles, inspect for lacerations, localized areas of edema, and ecchymoses that may indicate underlying injury. Care must be taken to adequately remove any debris and dried blood in this region, which can easily camouflage lacerations and lead to missed injuries.

Diligently assess cranial nerve function by specific provocative maneuvers. These injuries associated with lacerations are grossly identified by inspection of facial asymmetry at rest and during animation and by assessing sensory function (see Table 6–1 in Chapter 6).

Utilizing palpation, appreciate focal areas of tenderness, depressions, crepitus, and edema that may indicate hematoma or a bony fracture. Patients that have injuries suspicious of facial fractures should have their wounds débrided, closed, and referred for radiographic evaluation (see Chapter 6, Radiographic Evaluation section).

♦ Treatment

General Procedures

- Follow basic laceration closure procedures (see Chapter 3)
- Measure the laceration then irrigate, débride, initiate tetanus prophylaxis
- Always be aware of the consequences of your débridement. Débridement in some locations has little consequences; however, débridement around the nose, eyelids, and brow may lead to severe disfigurement.
- When patients present with severe "road rash" or a blast injury, clean the wound meticulously under loupe magnification. This procedure is time consuming, but you will have better results.
- Local anesthesia
    - Field blocks with 1% lidocaine/1:100,000 epinephrine through a 25- or 27-gauge needle
    - Consider regional blocks for large lacerations isolated to a single nerve distribution
    - Regional blocks of the trigeminal nerve are performed by instillation of 2 to 4 cc of local anesthesia (1% lidocaine or 0.25% Marcaine (Abbott Laboratories, Abbott Park, IL) just above the periosteum in the region of the nerve (**Fig. 7–1**).
    - Respect anatomical landmarks
- Close lacerations as soon as possible; waiting 2 or 3 days will compromise the results. To avoid depressed scarring, close deep tissue with the following sutures:
    - Muscle – Monocryl 4–0, Vicryl 4–0 (both by Ethicon, Somerville, NJ)
    - Skin
        - Deep layer – Monocryl 5–0, 6–0
        - Superficial layer – nylon/Prolene (Ethicon, Somerville, NJ) 6–0, 7–0
    - Mucosa – chromic 3–0, 4–0

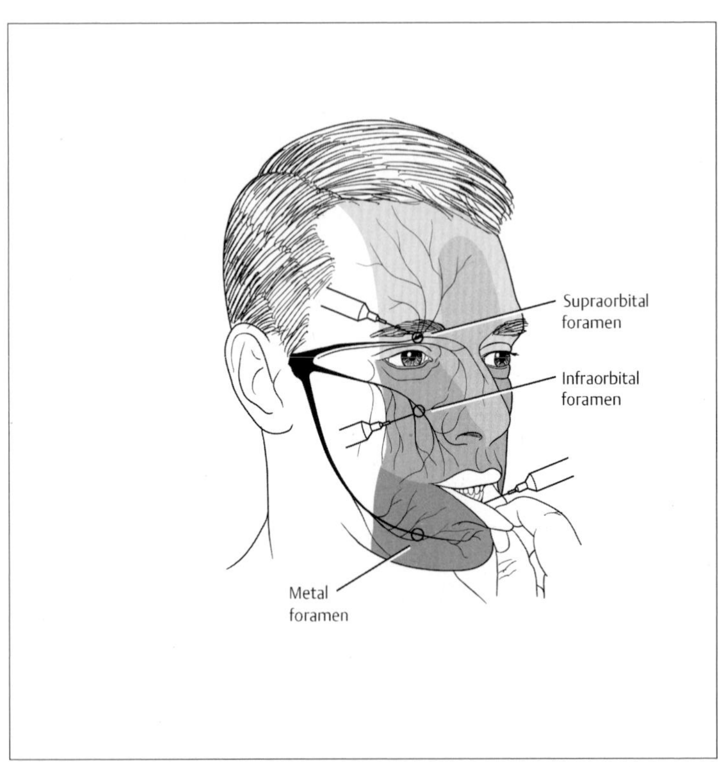

Figure 7–1 Placement procedures for regional blocks of the trigeminal nerve for the repair of facial soft tissue trauma.

- Manage superficial lacerations with minimal disfigurement conservatively
- Cleanse abrasions daily and apply antibiotic ointment (bacitracin t.i.d.)
- Close wound
  - Steri-Strip (3M, St. Paul, MN)
  - Dermabond (Ethicon, Somerville, NJ)

For pediatric patients:

- Pursue radiographic evaluation to rule out any associated fractures
- Conscious sedation (Chapter 2) to reduce emotional trauma for the patient and to repair difficult lacerations in specialized areas safely (e.g., periorbital region)

- Use absorbable sutures
  - Skin
    - Deep layer – Monocryl 5–0, 6–0
    - Superficial layer – fast-absorbing plain gut 5–0, 6–0
  - Mucosa – chromic 5–0
  - Muscle – 4–0 vicryl

Lip Lacerations

- Approximate each layer of a full-thickness laceration (**Fig. 7–2**)
  - Muscle – Monocryl 3–0, 4–0, Vicryl 3–0, 4–0
  - Skin – nylon/Prolene 6–0, 7–0
  - Mucosa (all surface of lip) – chromic 3–0, 4–0

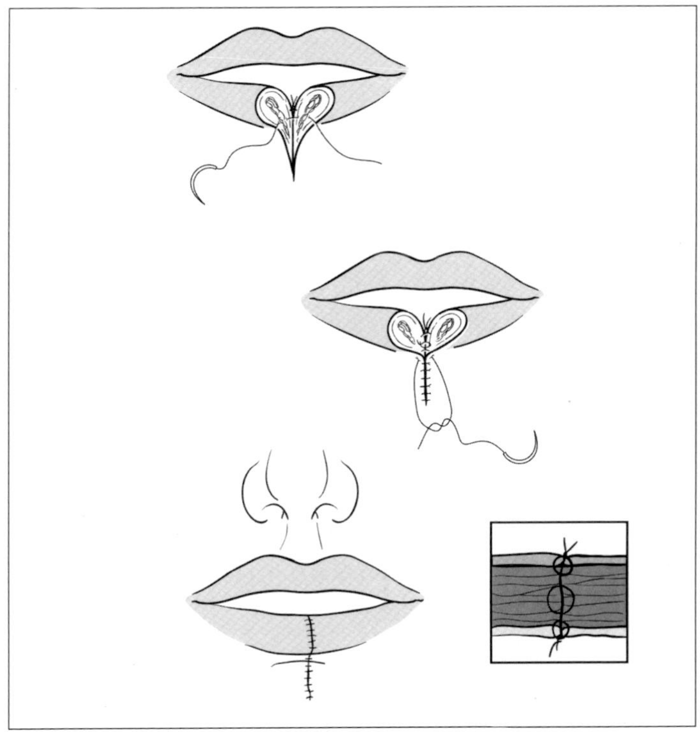

Figure 7–2 Layered closure of lip lacerations.

- Instruct the patient to minimize oral movement as much as possible for 5 days after repair.

Lacerations through the white roll (skin–vermilion border):

- Approximate the white roll exactly to obtain the best cosmetic outcome
- Align the white roll (vermillion–cutaneous junction), philtral columns, and cupids bow *before* injection with local anesthesia. These anatomical landmarks will be distorted by the edema that occurs after injection. Mark the vermillion for reapproximation *prior* to injecting the local anesthetic.
- The orbicularis oris is approximated at the appropriate height
- The skin is approximated with a nonabsorbable suture (nylon, Prolene 6–0) at the white roll
- Suture the vermillion with 5–0 chromic gut sutures

Ear Lacerations

- Irrigate ear lacerations thoroughly, but débride conservatively to prevent cartilage exposure
- Ensure skin closure over cartilage to avoid chondritis
- Approximate skin and perichondrium in a single bite using nonabsorbable sutures (Prolene, 6–0)
- Prescribe oral prophylactic antibiotics (Bactrim DS PO b.i.d. [Roche Pharmaceuticals, Nutley, NJ]) for 5 to 7 days.
- Clean and cover incisions twice a day with antibiotic ointment (Sulfamylon [Mylan Laboratories, Canonsburg, PA] or gentamicin ointment)
- Prepare dressings to avoid hematoma formation (**Fig. 6–5**)
- Apply Xeroform with fluffed gauze in a pressure dressing with circumferential head wrap
- Assess for perichondrial hematomas (Chapter 6)

Large Defects

Large defects with either composite or excessive skin loss may require secondary reconstructive procedures for closure (i.e., skin graft, partial composite resection).

- Cover ear with Xeroform and employ frequent dressing changes until reconstruction to avoid desiccation of the cartilage

Avulsion Injuries

- Treat immediately to avoid vascular compromise
- Débride, trim, and attach small avulsion fragments as a composite graft (<1.5 cm)

Amputation and large avulsions may require microvascular attachment depending on the site of avulsion and residual vasculature. Alternatively, the cartilage architecture may be preserved by dermabrasion of the avulsed part with storage under a postauricular flap or in the abdominal subcutaneous tissue ("pocket principle"). This will allow use of this fragment for delayed reconstruction. However, this procedure is not as optimal as reattachment of the ear, if reattachment is possible.

Venous congestion is a common problem after repair of avulsions. Large avulsed fragments and amputated ears will require leech therapy for survival.

Scalp Lacerations

- Rule out intracranial injury
- Promote hemostasis with a pressure dressing until the environment is appropriate for exploration
- Identify all lacerations by carefully removing debris and blood with hydrogen peroxide. Shaving is rarely necessary.
- Irrigate wounds with ample amounts of normal saline and remove any missed foreign bodies
- Layered closure
  - Galea – Vicryl, Monocryl 2–0
  - Skin – full-thickness bites, continuous suture for hemostasis – Prolene (blue) 3–0, 4–0, or staples
- Use smooth pickups to pull hair out from the wound and underneath the sutures
- Use Penrose cut longitudinally under scalp flap for wound drainage for 1–2 days

Eyelid and Eyebrow Lacerations

- Rule out ocular injuries (see Chapters 9 and 10)
- Beware of lacrimal duct injury
- Copious irrigation to remove ocular foreign bodies
- Layer by layer closure of conjunctiva, tarsus, and skin
  - Orbicularis – 6–0 Vicryl suture
  - Skin – 6–0 fast-absorbing gut or 6–0 nylon

For eyebrow lacerations:

- Do not shave
- Layered closure
  - Deep layer – Monocryl, Vicryl 5–0
  - Skin – exactly align brow elements – Prolene 5–0, 6–0

Eyelid Margin Lacerations (Fig. 7–3)

- Approximate lid margin
- Evert the lid margin to prevent lid notching with vertical mattress suture
- Antemarginal tarsus
  - Two or three 6–0 Vicryl sutures
  - One-half to three-quarters thickness tarsus

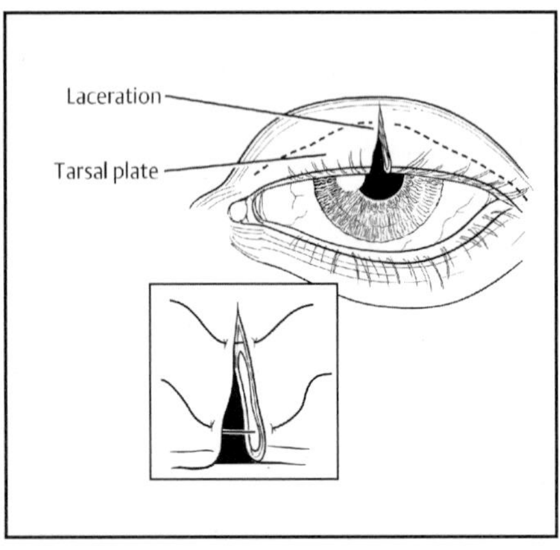

Figure 7–3 Repair of full-thickness eyelid laceration with repair of tarsus.

- Knot ends directed away from the cornea
- Skin – Prolene 7–0

Nasal Lacerations

- Achieve nasal hemostasis (see Chapter 10)
- Inspect nasal cavity to rule out nasal septal hematoma
  - Drain hematoma under direct vision with a 11-blade scalpel
- Layered closure of full-thickness lacerations
  - Mucosal layer – plain gut 4–0
  - Align skin and cartilage together with Prolene 6–0
- Splint nose with Steri-strips

Facial Hematomas

- Evaluate for intracranial injuries and C-spine injury
- Administer pain medication
- Apply cold compresses for 48 hours, and then apply warm compresses until resolution
- Drain hematomas that compromise the airway or visual axis
- Explore hematomas that are expanding despite adequate pressure therapy
- Evacuate hematomas that predispose the overlying skin to pressure necrosis
- When a hematoma is coupled with a laceration, use the laceration as an access point for evacuation
- Aspirate hematomas that occur in the malar region using an intraoral incision to avoid inflicting additional facial scars

♦ Facial Nerve Injuries

Lacerations through the submucosal aponeurotic system (SMAS) and musculature put the nerve at risk at any point along its route (**Fig. 7–4**).

- Injury to the temporal and zygomatic branches confers an inability to elevate the brow or close the eye, respectively.
- Damage to the buccal branch causes loss of the nasolabial crease and an inability to elevate the lip.

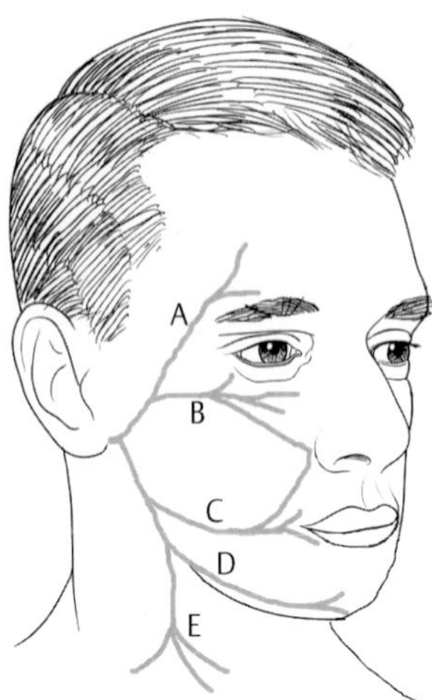

Figure 7–4 The course of the facial nerve. **(A)** Fronto-temporal branch, **(B)** zygomatic branch, **(C)** buccal branch, **(D)** marginal mandibular branch, and **(E)** cervical branch.

- Marginal mandibular nerve injury causes weakness of the lower lip depressors (frowning).

Facial nerve lacerations:

- Once identified, repair is begun within 72 hours. Repair within this time frame allows for the identification of severed nerve ends using a nerve stimulator before the motor end plates are depleted of neurotransmitters.
- Attempted repair after 72 hours is extraordinarily difficult secondary to contraction of the cut segment and the inability to stimulate the distal end for exact matching to the proximal end.
- Repair the nerve in the operating room under loupe magnification or with the microscope
- Identify and trim the proximal and distal nerve ends prior to anastomoses
- Anastomose the fresh nerve ends using tension-free 9–0 or 10–0 nonabsorbable (nylon) sutures in an epineural fashion
- Significant nerve loss or tension may require nerve grafting or the use of artificial nerve conduits.

Blunt injuries to the face that cause neuropraxia to the facial nerve:

- Do not require immediate operative measures
- Monitor for signs of improvement over the course of 3 weeks
- If there is no evidence of healing, refer the patient for electrodiagnostic testing (ENOG, EMG)
  - Identification of advanced architectural injury to the nerve at this point warrants exploration and repair.

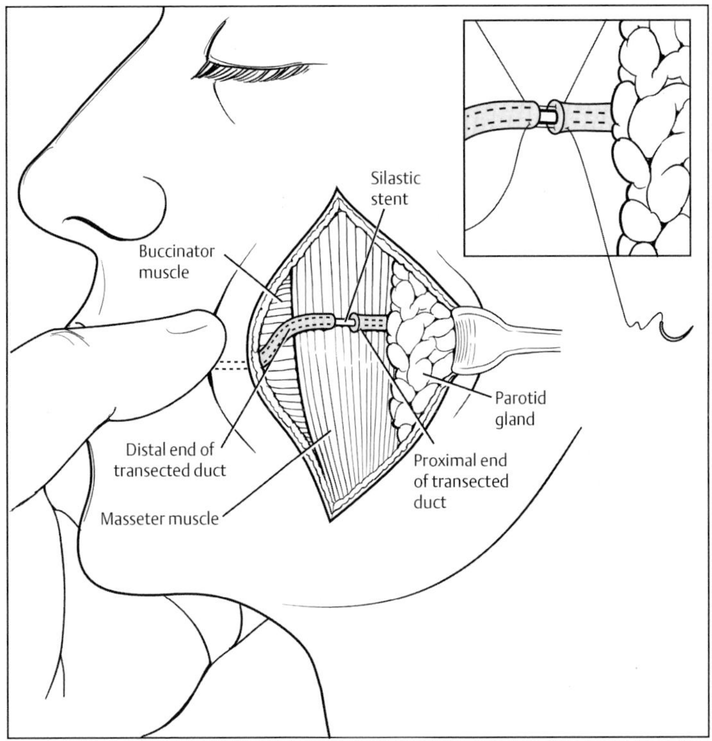

Figure 7–5 Repair of parotid duct injury over Silastic stent (Dow Corning, Midland, MI and Barry, UK).

♦ Parotid Duct Injuries

The parotid duct traverses in a plane from the tragus to the middle of the upper lip. The duct orifice is in the buccal mucosa opposite the second maxillary molar. Extraoral or intraoral lacerations place these structures at risk for injury. Injury to the buccal branch of the facial nerve should also raise suspicion for parotid duct injury. A patient with a suspected parotid duct laceration can be tested easily by placing toothpaste in the patient's oral cavity. Excessive saliva will be expressed from the laceration.

- Evaluate a parotid duct injury by cannulating the intraoral segment with a 22-gauge Angiocath (BD Medical, Sandy UT).
- Inject 1 cc of milk or methylene blue (messy) to assess patency.
- Repair lacerated duct over a stent in the operating room using 7–0 monofilament sutures inylon (**Fig. 7–5**).
- Keep the stent in place for 5 days to allow patency and prevent fistula formation.
- Give the patient prophylactic antibiotics during this period.
- Reconstruct ostia for the proximal segment or duct ligation if there is severe irreparable damage of the parotid duct.
- Oversew parotid gland injuries without duct injuries with absorbable suture – Monocryl 3.0, 4.0, vicryl.

8

Orbit and Zygoma Fractures

♦ The Orbit

Anatomy

The orbit is composed of seven bones:

- Zygoma
- Greater and lesser wing of the sphenoid
- Ethmoid
- Frontal
- Palatine
- Maxilla
- Lacrimal

These seven bones create a bony pyramid with the optic canal at the apex. The orbit is comprised of the following structures

- Floor
- Roof of the maxillary sinus
- Medial wall
- Lamina papyracea of the ethmoid bone
- Lacrimal bone
- Lateral wall
- Zygoma and greater wing of the sphenoid bone
- Roof
- Frontal bone – floor of the frontal sinus

The medial wall is the weakest structure, followed by the floor. The roof and the lateral wall are generally the strongest. The optic nerve exits the optic canal situated superomedially and ~40 to 45 mm from the inferior orbital rim. The superior orbital fissure separates the greater and lesser wings of the sphenoid. From the superior orbital fissure traverses the

- Oculomotor nerve (CN III)
- Trochlear nerve (CN IV)
- Abducens nerve (CN VI)
- Ophthalmic division of the trigeminal nerve (CN V_1)

The inferior orbital fissure provides passage of the

- Maxillary division of trigeminal (CN V_2)
- Branches of sphenopalatine ganglion
- Branches of the inferior ophthalmic vein

Physical Examination

Orbital fractures are usually associated with blunt trauma. Nearly 30% of orbital fractures will have injuries to the globe. It is important to perform a detailed ophthalmic exam that includes visual acuity, pupillary reaction, retinal exam, and red color saturation, as described in Chapter 7. Any deviation from normal warrants an emergent ophthalmic consultation.

Pathologic physical findings include

- Orbital ecchymosis
- Periorbital edema
- Subconjunctival hemorrhage
- Epistaxis
- Orbital rim/zygoma bony step-offs
- Diplopia
- Extraocular muscle entrapment
  - Examine the active range of motion of the extraocular muscles to rule out mechanical entrapment.
  - In unconscious patients, perform the forced duction test: using Adson forceps grasp the inferior capsulopalpebral fascia of

the inferior rectus muscle and gently rotate the globe, while feeling for any restrictions.

- Intraorbital edema
- Optic nerve neuropraxia
- Pupillary shape – oblong pupil is suggestive of ocular perforation
- Pupillary response – afferent pupillary defect (see Chapter 7)
- Supraorbital, infraorbital, alveolar nerve paresthesias
- Crepitus/subcutaneous emphysema – disruption of maxillary or ethmoid sinus mucosa
- Enophthalmos – noticeably with >2 mm shift; however, rarely evident immediately postinjury because of edema
- Proptosis/exophthalmos
- Hyphema – fluid in the anterior chamber of the eye
- Superior orbital fissure (SOF) syndrome – fractures of the SOF result in
    - Fixed dilated pupil (CN III)
    - Upper lid ptosis (CN III)
    - Loss of corneal reflex (CN V1)
    - Ophthalmoplegia (CN IV, CN VI)
- Orbital apex syndrome – SOF syndrome plus impairment of optic nerve as it exists in the optic canal
- Nausea, vomiting, bradycardia – oculocardiac response to extraocular muscle entrapment (**Fig. 8–1**)

Treatment

Patients suspected of having acute compressive optic neuropathy should undergo emergent decompression. Decompression is performed with a lateral canthotomy or by fracturing the medial orbital floor. Start methylprednisolone (load 30 mg/kg followed in 2 hours by 15 mg/kg q6h), acetazolamide (250 mg PO b.i.d.), and mannitol (1 g/kg IV, repeat q6h PRN).

To perform a lateral canthotomy, retract the upper and lower lid superiorly and inferiorly, respectively, with your index and third finger. Incise the lateral canthal skin 4 to 5 mm, then palpate the lateral canthal tendon with fine scissors and release overlying soft tissue lateral to the conjunctiva all the way down to the lateral

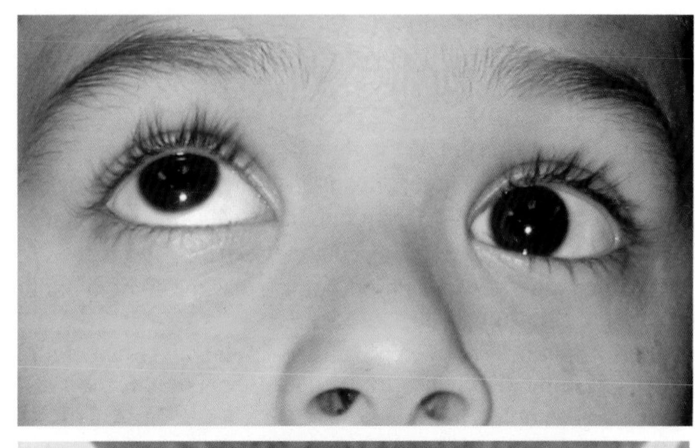

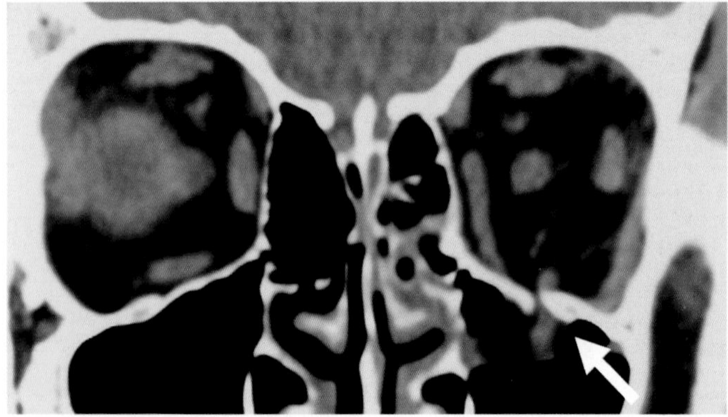

Figures 8–1 (A,B) Diplopia associated with entrapment of the inferior rectus muscle limiting ocular mobility. **(B)** Arrow indicates trapdoor.

bony orbit. Disinsertion of the canthal tendon will result in a more freely mobile eye along with complete mobility of the lower lid.

To fracture the medial orbital floor, first manually retract the lower lid. With a pair of fine hemostats, push through the floor medially to allow drainage into the maxillary sinus.

A subset of patients with ocular injuries will present with vision loss secondary to optic nerve trauma (compression or edema) without increased extraocular orbital pressure. These patients are suspected of having traumatic optic neuropathy. The etiology may be direct secondary to bony fragments within the optic canal. Indirect injury is secondary to ischemia and edema of the optic nerve. Emergent high-resolution CT of the orbit is performed to identify specific anatomical optic nerve pathology. Patients with decreased light perception should be started on a megadose of steroids for 48 hours (methylprednisolone load 30 mg/kg followed in 2 hours by 15 mg/kg q6h). Patients that exhibit worsening light perception or that present with no light perception should be considered for operative optic nerve decompression.

Types of Orbital Fractures

Orbital fractures can occur anywhere along the medial or lateral walls, floor, roof, and apex. Most commonly, they will be localized to the medial wall and floor, the weakest structures. Medial wall fractures are part of a complex of fractures associated with the nasal and ethmoid bones; they are discussed in Chapter 10.

Orbital Floor

Orbital floor fractures (blow out) are the second most common midface fractures behind nasal fractures. Fractures most commonly occur at the medial wall and floor of the orbit along the infraorbital groove (paresthesia). A fracture defect may entrap periorbital fat and possibly the inferior rectus muscle (**Fig. 8–2**). The pathomechanics of the injury include two theories:

1 The hydraulic theory – direct trauma to the globe leads to increased intraorbital pressure resulting in a decompressing fracture at the weakest point.

2 The bone conduction theory – an indirect transmission of forces around the orbital rim leading to fracture of the floor.

Orbital Roof

Fractures to the orbital roof are rare due to protection by the supraorbital rim and strong frontal bone. These fractures are more common in children secondary to the differences in the architecture of the cranium. When fractures in the roof occur, displacement can be either into the anterior cranial fossa or more commonly into the orbit causing a "blow-in" fracture. Evaluation of these patients by CT should rule out both intracranial and intraocular involvement. Blow-in fractures are characterized by a decreased orbital volume (i.e., exophthalmos), and commonly warrant urgent surgical intervention to

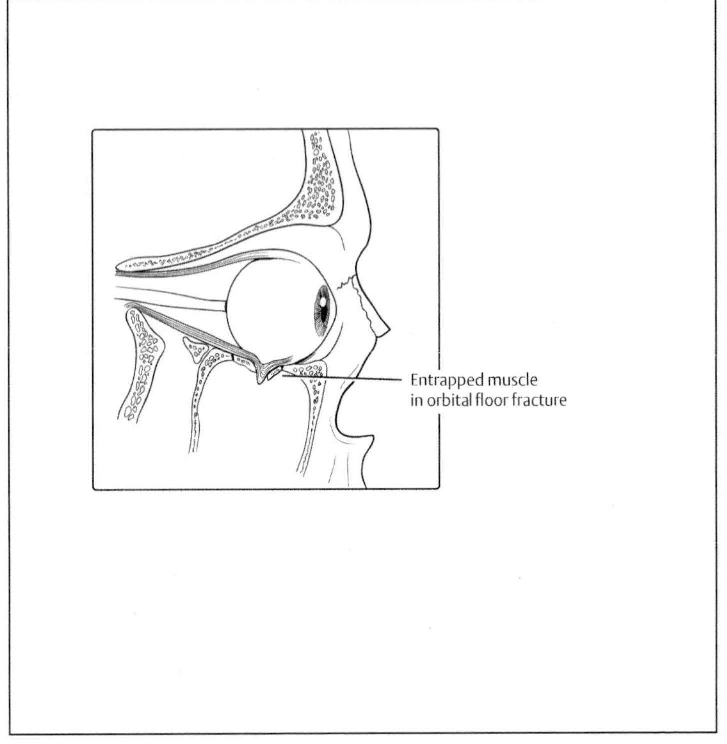

Figure 8–2 Incomplete orbital floor fracture with entrapment of inferior rectus.

decrease the increased intraocular pressure. Additionally, injury to the supraorbital artery can result in a retrobulbar hematoma.

Radiographic Evaluation

CT scans should be obtained with 1.5-mm thin cuts through the orbit with sagittal and coronal reconstructions. Evaluate the scans for

- Displaced fracture fragments
  - Trapdoor fracture
  - Bony fragment impingement on optic canal

- Area of floor defect
- Soft tissue entrapment
- Enophthalmos
- Lens dislocation
- Retrobulbar hematoma
- Other associated fractures (medial wall fracture)

Surgical Indications

Surgical indications include

- Early enophthalmos >2 mm (6 weeks)
- Symptomatic diplopia >2 weeks (primary field)
- Displaced fracture with floor defect >1 cm^2
- Hypoglobus – low vertical lying globe
- Positive forced duction test
- Oculocardiac response –bradycardia, nausea, syncope

Management

Patients without any of the surgical indications listed above or any signs of globe injury can be discharged home. Nondisplaced fractures will commonly be associated with early enophthalmos and diplopia, both of which are not urgent surgical indications. Patients should be followed closely for 2 weeks to ensure resolution of symptoms. Pain medication should be prescribed as indicated; antibiotics are not indicated. Patients should be instructed to use artificial tears to keep the eye lubricated and to minimize nose blowing to avoid orbital emphysema and displacement of a fracture.

Patients that do require surgical intervention should be seen by an ophthalmologist prior to surgery to rule out open globe injuries. Fractures are optimally operated on within 24 hours (before significant edema develops) or after 2 weeks (once edema resolves).

Emergent surgery includes those patients who have clear bony displacement into the optic canal or globe as confirmed by CT, or signs and symptoms suggestive of oculocardiac response.

♦ Zygoma/Zygomatico Maxillary Complex Fractures

The zygoma articulates with the frontal, sphenoid, maxillary, and temporal bone comprising the characteristic tetrapod (**Fig. 8–3**). It is composed of two faces, the malar face, which comprises the lateral orbit, and the body, which gives projection to the cheek. The zygomatic process of the temporal bone articulates with the body of the zygoma to create the zygomatic arch. The zygoma has multiple muscular attachments; most important is the masseter, which produces a major inferior deforming force on the body and arch when fractured. Fractures and disarticulations of the zygoma usually

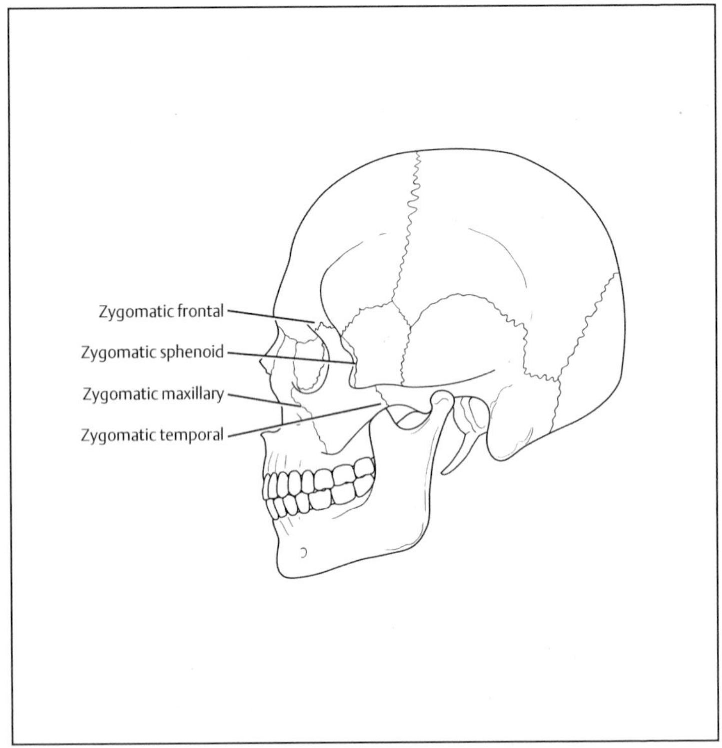

Figure 8–3 Zygomatic tetraploid bone articulations.

result in an inferior displacement, leading to increased intraorbital volume producing enophthalmos. These fractures are most commonly referred to as tripod or a zygomaticomaxillary complex (ZMC) fracture, so called because it involves separation of all four major attachments of the zygoma to the rest of the face. Occasionally, however, there can be an isolated fracture of the zygomatic arch or lateral wall without concomitant ZMC fracture.

Symptoms and Physical Findings

- Enophthalmus
- Flattening of the midface / malar asymmetry
- Diplopia
- Trismus
- Impingement on coronoid process
- Periorbital and subconjunctival hematoma
  - "Flame sign"
- Epistaxis
- Inferior displacement of globe
- Inferior displacement of lateral canthus
- Infraorbital nerve injury – paresthesia of cheek, upper lip, anterior incisors, and alar of the nose
- Occlusion and range of motion disturbances
- Intraoral hematoma

Radiographic Evaluation

- Caldwell view
- Submental vertex
- Waters view
  - Most helpful plain film
  - 30 Degrees of occipitomental projection
  - Visualization of zygomatic buttresses
- CT
  - Axial
  - 1.5 mm
  - Coronal

- Orbital evaluation
- Reconstructions
  - 3D reconstructions

Management

Patients with nondisplaced ZMC fractures can be discharged home, observed, and treated conservatively. Antibiotics are not indicated. Keep patients on a soft diet (non-chew) for 6 weeks with protection of the malar eminence. Follow-up should be in 2 weeks to assess for displacement and enophthalmos. This can occur long term with masseter pull on the fractured zygoma.

Patients with displaced ZMC fractures should be prepared for surgery to realign the lateral orbital wall and floor and to correct contour irregularities of the malar eminence. An ophthalmologist's evaluation is warranted with orbital involvement.

Patients with nondisplaced isolated zygomatic arch fractures require no surgical intervention. They can be discharged home with malar eminence protection. Displaced isolated zygomatic fractures do not need admission and can be discharged home to have their fracture repaired electively. Repair is within 24 hours or delayed for 2 weeks after edema resolves.

Those patients with trismus secondary to impingement to the coronoid or masseter and cosmetic temporal deformities also warrant consideration for operative reduction.

9

Nasal and Nasal–Orbital–Ethmoid (NOE) Fractures

♦ Anatomy

The nasal area includes (**Fig. 9–1**)

- Nasal bone
- Frontal processes of the maxilla
- Nasal cartilages
- Nasal septum
- Quadrilateral cartilage
- Perpendicular plate of the ethmoid
- Vomer

Blood supply:

- Ophthalmic artery is the first branch of the internal carotid
- Anterior and posterior ethmoidal branches of internal carotid
- Facial artery branches
- Superior labial
- Internal maxillary branches of external carotid (sphenopalatine, greater palatine, and infraorbital)

External innervation:

- Nasociliary nerve V_1
- Supratrochlear nerve V_1
- Infraorbital nerve V_2

Internal innervation:

- Anterior ethmoid nerve V_1
- Greater palatine nerve - lateral wall
- Nasopalatine nerve V_2

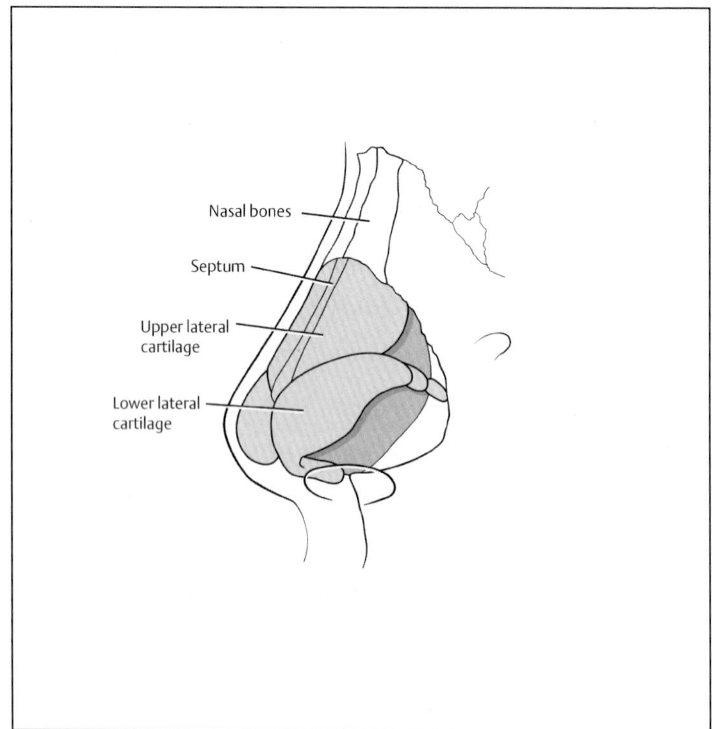

Figure 9–1 (A) Bony and cartilaginous vault anatomy.

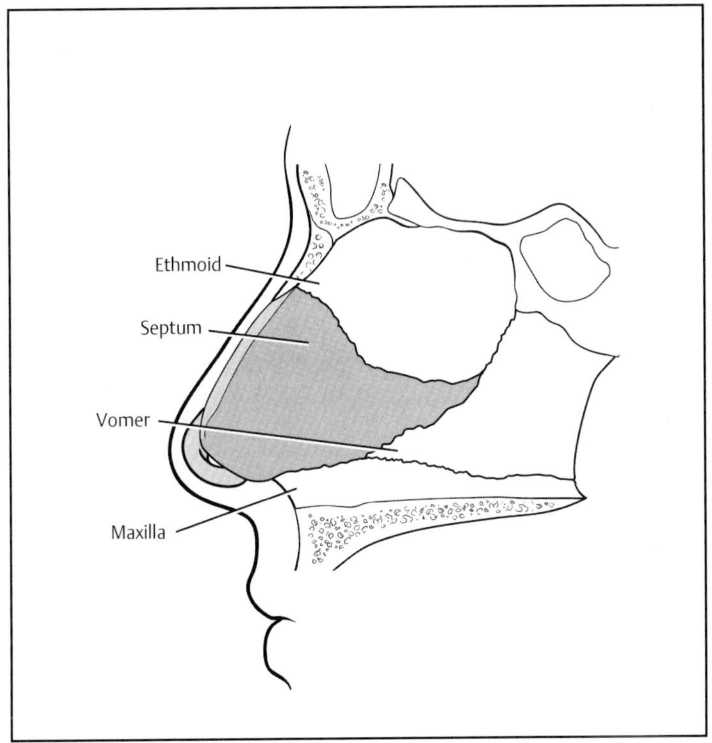

Figure 9–1 *(Continued)* **(B)** Nasal septal anatomy.

♦ Nasal Fractures

Physical Examination

Nasal fractures are usually a result of blunt trauma directly to the nose. Evaluation of the nose should take place in a well-lighted area with the patient comfortably seated and reclined at a 45-degree angle to facilitate inspection of both the external and internal nasal cavity. Suction, irrigation, nasal speculum, head light/hand-held light, and cotton-tip applicators should be readily available. Common physical findings include

- Tenderness
- Crepitus
- Nasal deviation

- Mobility
- Epistaxis
- Airway obstruction
- Septal deviation
- Septal hematoma
- Saddle deformity
- Mucosal laceration

Septal Hematomas

Septal hematomas are caused by bleeding between the septum and mucosa. Diagnosis is made by direct visualization of a hematoma beneath the mucosa. Septal hematomas require immediate drainage and care in the acute setting. If left undrained, the accumulation of blood in the mucoperichondrium can lead to septal ischemia with potential septal necrosis. Complications include perforation, loss of dorsal support, and saddle deformity. Nasal septal hematomas should be drained appropriately with the proper pressure dressing applied (see Chapter 6, Fig. 6–4A). Packing should be removed on Day 3 to prevent sinusitis or toxic shock. Place patient on antibiotics.

Radiographic Evaluation

Plain films and CT scans (**Fig. 9–2**) are not absolutely necessary. Their necessity becomes more relevant if other injuries are

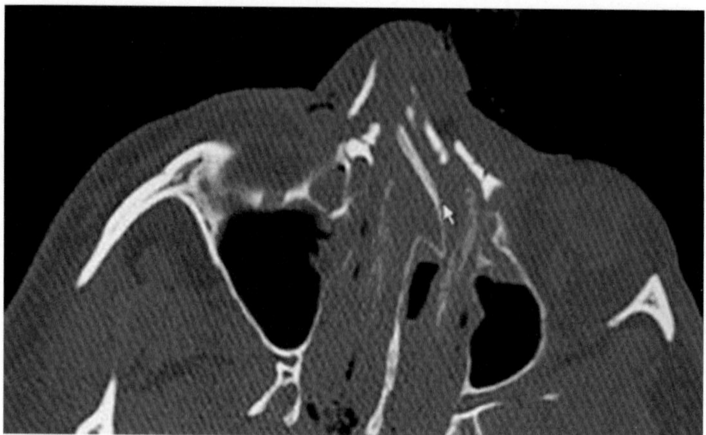

Figure 9–2 CT scan of nasal bone and septal fracture with orbital component.

suspected (e.g., nasal-orbital-ethmoid fractures [NOE], orbital floor fracture, intracranial bleed). If one has a low clinical suspicion for any other injury, nasal fractures in general do not require any radiography. In selected clinical scenarios, a nasal series (anterior and lateral view) can be ordered to aid in diagnosis and for documentation.

Stranc-Robertson Nasal Fracture Classification (Fig. 9–3)

- Type I
  - Anterior portion of the nasal pyramid
  - Septum

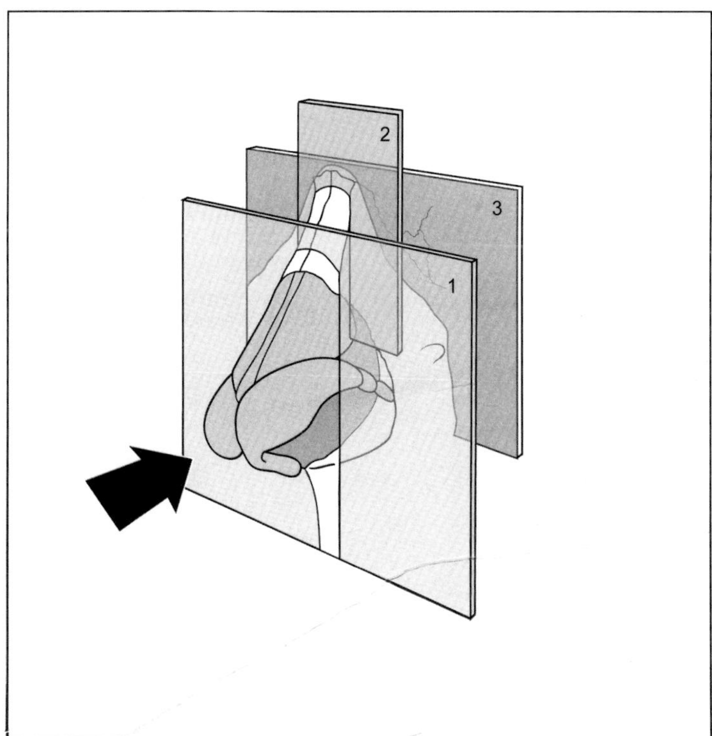

Figure 9–3 Stranc–Robertson nasal fracture classification.

- Type II
  - Comminution of the nasal pyramid
  - Dislocation of the septum
- Type III
  - Frontal processes of the maxilla
  - NOE fractures

Nasal Fracture Treatment

The timing of the repair is usually bimodal and correlated with the amount of edema. Any repair should be performed within the first 2 hours before the onset of significant edema. This is rarely the case when a patient presents and typically, repairs are usually performed after 1 to 2 weeks when the edema subsides.

Closed Reduction

Adequate anesthesia can be achieved locally if a reduction is attempted in the emergency care setting. Epinephrine 1:100,000 or 4% cocaine-soaked Cottonoid (Codman & Shurtleff, Raynham, MA)/pledgets or Afrin Spray (Schering-Plough Corp., Kenilworth, NJ) Cottonoid/pledgets applied intranasally for 5 minutes.

A regional block – 1% lidocaine with 0.25% Marcaine (Abbott Laboratories, Abbott Park, IL) mixed 1:1 provides long lasting pain relief with fast onset. Epinephrine can also be added at 1:100,000.

- Regional block (see Chapter 7, Fig. 7–1)
  - Nasociliary nerve
  - Infratrochlear nerve
  - Infraorbital nerves
  - Tip – columella

Asch or Walsham forceps can be used to realign and reduce the fracture (**Fig. 9–4**). The blunt end of a scalpel handle can also be used. Reduction should be aimed at repositioning the nose to the midline. Reshaping the nasal pyramid often involves "outfracturing" of the nasal sidewalls. Assess reduction by visualization and palpation.

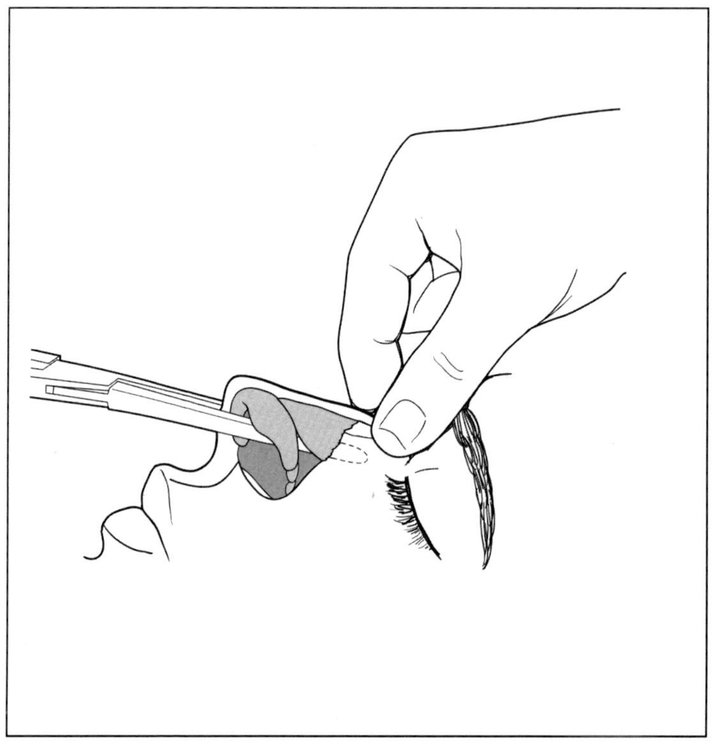

Figure 9–4 Closed reduction of nasal fracture using Walsham forceps.

♦ Postreduction Care

- Packing – place packing in distinct layers, if necessary to achieve hemostasis (see Chapter 6, Fig. 6–4.)
  - Merocel (Merocel Surgical Products, Mystic, CT), Xeroform gauze, Vaseline (Unilever PLC, Englewood Cliffs, NJ)/bacitracin impregnated gauze, Cottonoid soaked with epinephrine 1:100,000.
  - Remove packing within 3 days to avoid sinusitis or toxic shock (see Chapter 6, Fig. 6–4A).
  - Prescribe antibiotics for patients with intranasal packing
    - Augmentin (GlaxoSmithKline, Mississauga, Ontario, Canada) 875 mg PO b.i.d. × 3 days, or
    - Clindamycin 450 mg PO q.i.d. × 3 days

- Splint – apply an external nasal splint to the dorsum (**Fig. 9–5**); keep splints in place for 7 to 10 days.
  - Fashion a splint out of a small piece of plaster over steri-strips if prefabricated thermoplastic splints are not available
- No nose blowing for several weeks
- No contact to nose
- Follow-up within one week

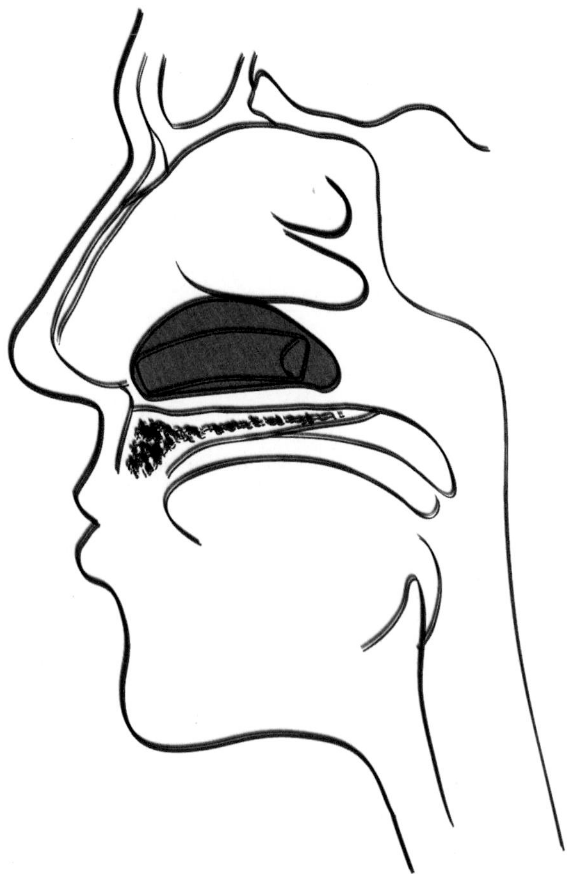

Figure 9–5 Postreduction intracranial/nasal splint

Nasal fractures that are significantly displaced or with significant edema not facilitating reduction in the acute setting can be discharged home with contact precautions. Antibiotics are not needed, and patients should follow up in 2 weeks for attempted closed or open operative reduction.

♦ Nasal-Orbital-Ethmoid Fractures

NOE fractures result from blunt force directly over the nasal pyramid. The nose is depressed between the orbits resulting in fractures of the nasal bone and medial orbital wall. Fractures are commonly bilateral, but one third of the time they are unilateral. The high forced impact will often be accompanied with orbital blowout fractures as well.

Anatomy

The anatomy includes

- Posterior
  - Sphenoid bone
- Roof
  - Anterior cranial fossa
- Lateral extension of interorbital space
  - Medial orbital walls
- Anterior structures
  - Maxilla, frontal and nasal bones

The medial canthal ligament is the direct extension of the orbicularis oculi muscle with insertion onto medial orbital wall. The ligament is comprised of three limbs, which help provide medial support to the globe along with keeping the eyelids tangential to the globe. The superior, anterior, and posterior limbs together form a tent that houses the lacrimal sac. This ligament is important in the classification of NOE fractures.

Physical Examination

- Loss of dorsal-nasal prominence (saddle deformity)
- Glabellar, periorbital, nasal ecchymosis
- Bony crepitus over canthal region
- Telecanthus ≥ 35 mm (normal 30 to 32 mm)
- Bowstring test – lateral traction of lower eyelid will result in telecanthus if ligament is disrupted
- Rhinorrhea – indication of a cribriform plate fracture
- Olfactory disturbance

Radiographic Evaluation

- CT scan – 1.5-mm cuts axial and coronal

Markowitz Classification (Fig. 9–6)

- Type I – single segment central fracture with medial canthal tendon attached
- Type II – comminuted fracture with medial canthal tendon attached
- Type III – comminuted fracture with avulsed medial canthal tendon

Treatment and Management

Patients with NOE fractures need to be admitted and monitored, and contaminated intracranial injury should be ruled out. Urgent ophthalmology evaluation is warranted to rule out injury to the globe. The patient should be assessed for leakage of cerebrospinal fluid (CSF), which may indicate damage to the cribriform plate, frontal sinus, or anterior cranial fossa. CSF rhinorrhea is evaluated by performing the Halo test: formation of a halo when CSF placed on tissue paper, or by laboratory analysis of glucose or β-transferrin in the nasal drainage. If potential dural contamination is suspected, a neurosurgical consult is appropriate.

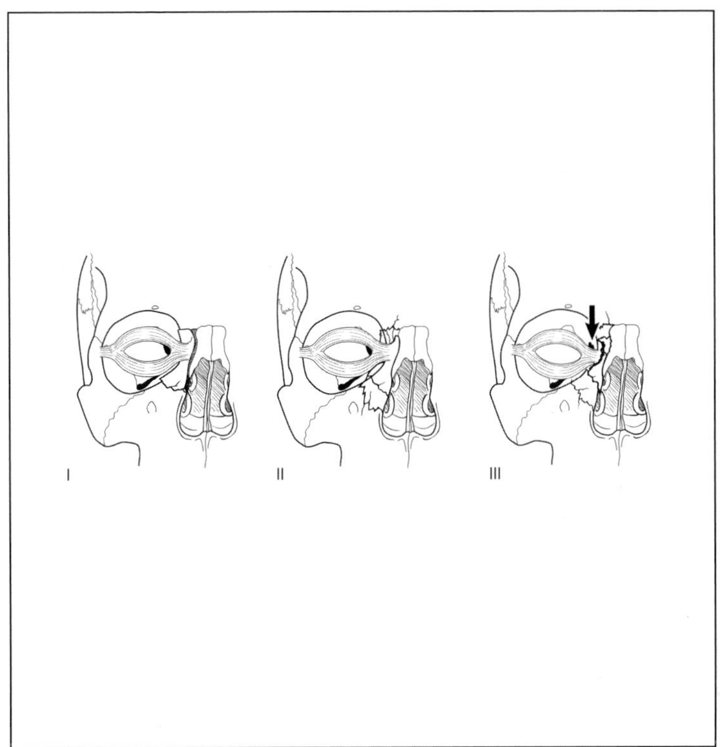

Figure 9–6 Markowitz classification of nasal-orbital-ethmoid fractures.

- Place patient on IV antibiotics (Clindamycin 600 IV q6h, Rocephin 1 gm IV q24h (Roche Pharmaceuticals, Nutley, NJ)
- Fractures will likely be explored and repaired.
- Elevate head of bed
- No nose blowing
- Follow appropriate preoperative procedures (NPO, IV fluids, etc.) if surgery is planned

10

Frontal Sinus Fractures

The frontal bone is the strongest bone of the face; a direct isolated high-energy impact is usually needed to fracture this bone. The frontal sinuses are absent in 4% of individuals, rudimentarily developed in 5%, and unilateral in 10% of individuals.

♦ Anatomy

The anatomy of the frontal sinuses is comprised of (**Fig. 10–1**)

- Two paired irregular cavities
- Anterior wall = anterior table
- Posterior wall = posterior table

♦ Physical Examination

- Forehead contusion
- Forehead laceration
- Forehead or orbital hematomas
- Epistaxis
- Otorrhea or rhinorrhea from dural tears – test with halo sign on paper towel; send fluid for glucose and β transfer
- Palpable step deformity secondary to underlying fracture; may be obscured by overlying swelling in the acute setting
- Paresthesias in the supraorbital nerve distribution

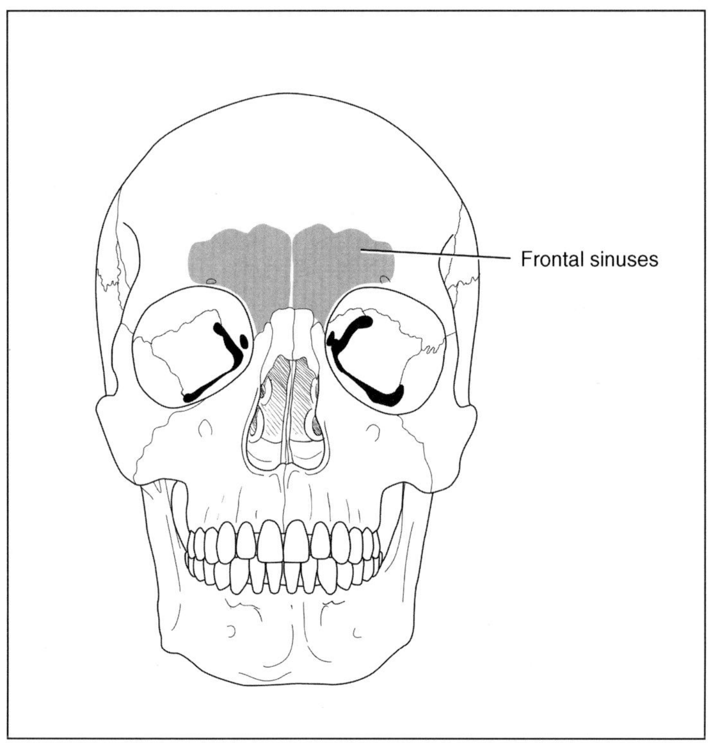

Figure 10–1 The frontal sinuses.

- Extension into the supraorbital rim and superior orbital fissure can lead to superior orbital fissure syndrome (see Chapter 8).
- Perform a thorough ocular exam

Radiographic Evaluation

CT of the face with 3-mm axial cuts and coronal reconstructions is the most sensitive modality for diagnosing frontal sinus fractures. Management will often be dependent on whether or not there is a nasofrontal duct injury. Fractures that are located inferiorly and medially should raise a high suspicion for nasofrontal duct injury (**Fig. 10–2; Fig. 10–3**).

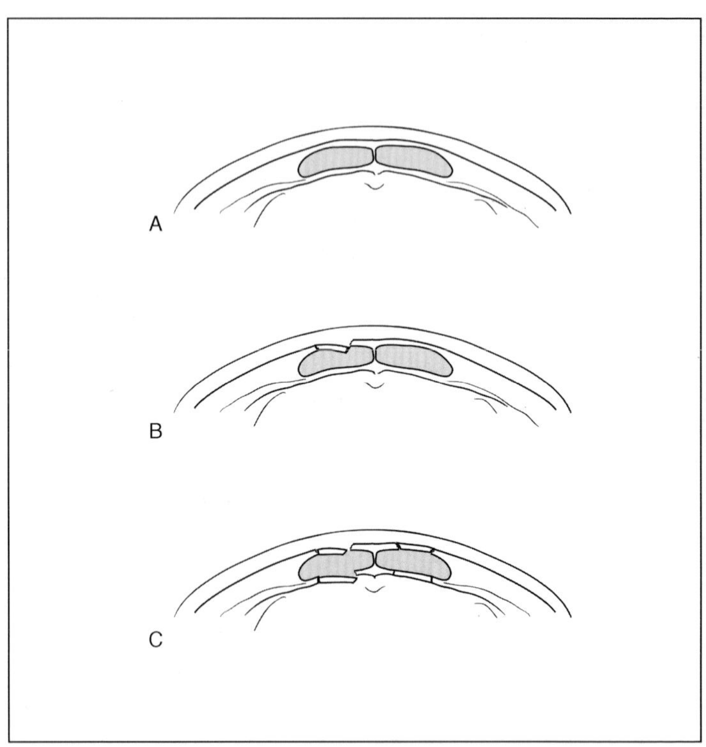

Figure 10–2 Frontal sinus fracture patterns. **(A)** Normal relationship. **(B)** Anterior table. **(C)** Comminuted anterior and posterior table.

♦ Management

All patients with frontal sinus fractures should be admitted and observed.

- Rule out
  - Subarachnoid hemorrhages
  - Subdural hematomas
  - Epidural hematomas
  - Cerebral contusions
  - Pneumocephalus

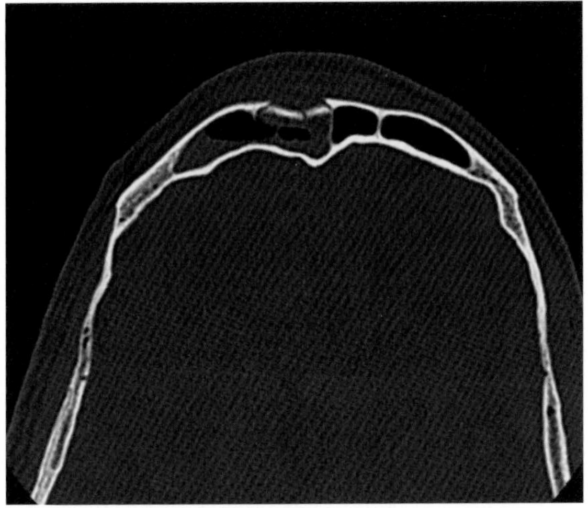

Figure 10–3 CT of anterior table fracture.

- No nose blowing
- Cough and sneeze with mouth open and not through nose
- Elevate head of bed to minimize edema
- Intravenous antibiotics
- Ceftriaxone 1 to 2 g IV q24h

Operative management is dependant on degree of fracture displacement, nasofrontal duct involvement, and dural integrity. Anterior table fractures induce cosmetic deformity and functional morbidity if the nasofrontal duct is involved. Obliteration of the nasofrontal duct is indicated when involved in the fracture line. Otherwise displaced fractures may by reduced and fixed in a delayed fashion.

Posterior table fractures occur in combination with anterior table fractures and presume the same sequela with the addition of the potential for anterior cranial fossa involvement and dural penetration. CSF leak is evident when the patient presents with significant rhinorrhea that is positive for β2 transferrin or creates a

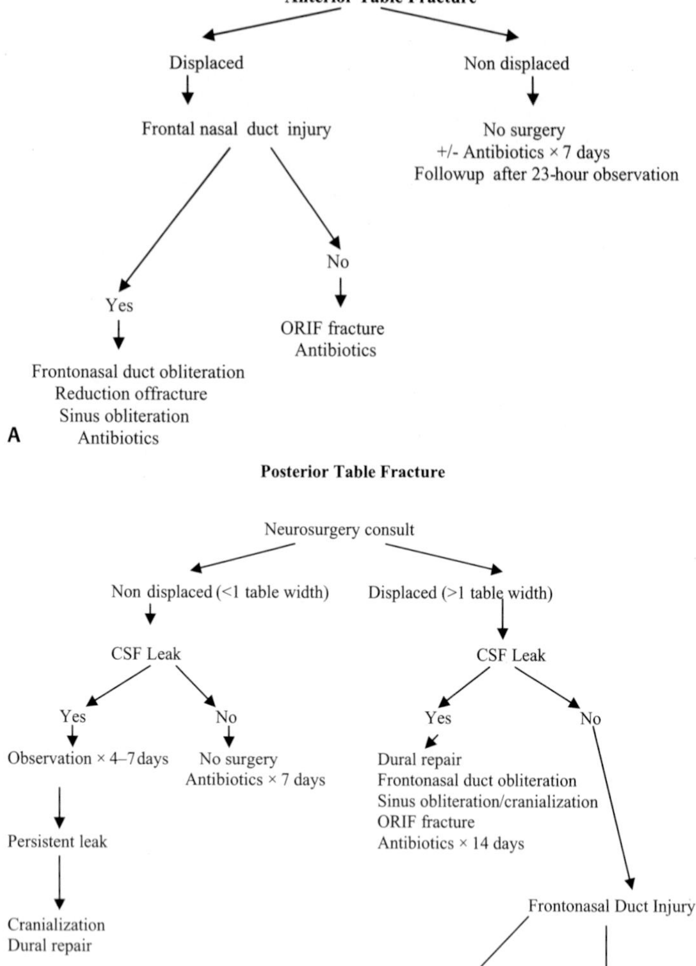

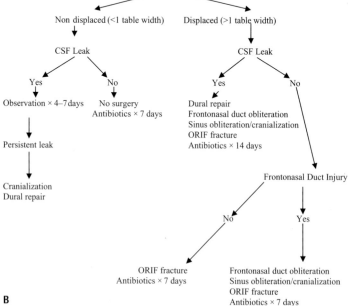

Figure 10–4(A) Algorithm for anterior table fracture **(B)** Algorithm for posterior table fracture

yellow ring on tissue paper (Halo test). If the posterior table is not displaced, the patient is observed for 4 to 7 days. Patients with persistent leakage of CSF fluid or displacement and comminution of the posterior table require cranialization. Specific fracture management strategies are outlined in **Fig. 10–4**.

11
Mandibular Fractures

♦ Anatomy

- A "U-" shaped bone that contains two hemimandibles
- Structures unite at midline called symphysis
- Each hemimandible consists of a (**Fig. 11–1**)
  - Body
  - Angle
  - Ramus
  - Coronoid process
  - Condyle
- Muscles of mastication
  - Jaw protrusion
    - Lateral pterygoid (lateral pterygoid plate to condylar neck)
  - Jaw elevators
    - Temporalis (temporal fossa to coronoid)
    - Masseter (zygomatic arch to the body)
    - Medial pterygoid (medial pterygoid plate to angle)
  - Jaw depressor-retractors
    - Lateral pterygoid
    - Digastric
    - Geniohyoid
    - Mylohyoid
    - Genioglossus

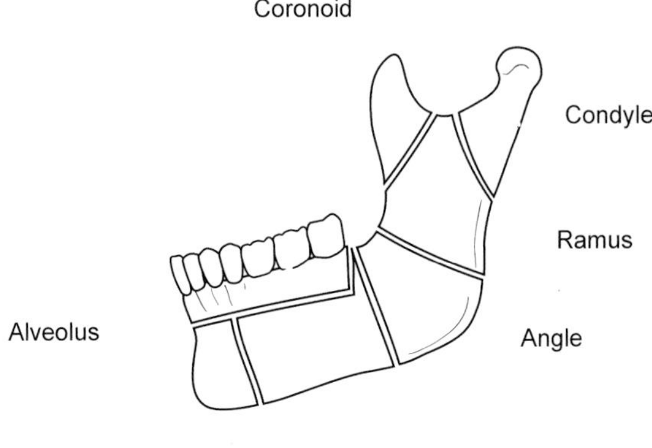

Figure 11–1 Anatomy of the mandible.

- Condyle articulates with cranium at the glenoid fossa of the temporomandibular joint (TMJ)
- Blood supply of mandible
  - Inferior alveolar artery from the internal maxillary artery enters at mandibular foramen and exits at mental foramen
  - Branches from the muscles of mastication
- Nerve supply
  - Inferior alveolar nerve from V_3 enters at mandibular foramen and exits at mental foramen
- Mental foramen
  - Located between first and second premolar

♦ Dental Relationships

Child:

- 20 deciduous or primary teeth labeled A – T
  - Right A B C D E F G H I J
  - Left T S R Q P O N M L K

Adult:

- 32 permanent teeth labeled 1 through 32

- Numbering begins with the third right maxillary molar as tooth #1 and the last maxillary molar as #16
- Numbering continues onto the mandibular left third molar as #17 and ends with the mandibular right third molar as #32

Each hemimandible or hemimaxilla consists of

- One central and one lateral incisor
- One canine (cuspid)
- First and second premolar (bicuspid)
- First, second, and third molar

Angle Classification of Occlusion

Based on the first maxillary molar and its position to the first mandibular molar (**Fig. 11–2**):

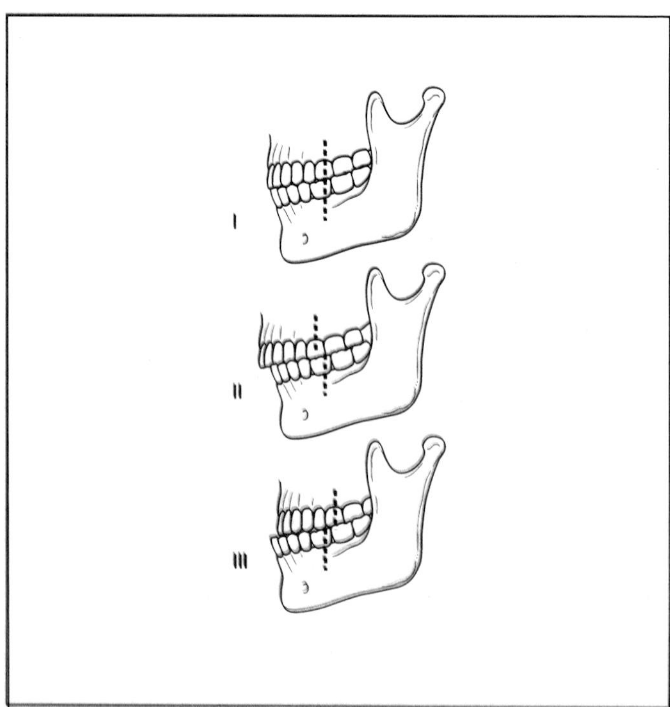

Figure 11–2 Angle classification of occlusion.

- Class I – normal occlusion
    - Mesiobuccal cusp of the maxillary first molar occludes with buccal groove of the mandibular first molar
- Class II – overbite
    - Lower first molar is distal (posterior) to the upper first molar
- Class III – underbite
    - Lower first molar is mesial (anterior) to the upper first molar

♦ Mandibular Fractures

Fractures of the mandible are often the result of physical altercations and have the highest frequency in men in the 25 to 34 age group. Fractures commonly arise in the thinnest portions of the bone in the angle and condylar region. The thick ramus is fractured the least often (**Fig. 11–3**). Mandibular fractures often transpire at two sites on the mandible due to the coup–contrecoup phenomenon.

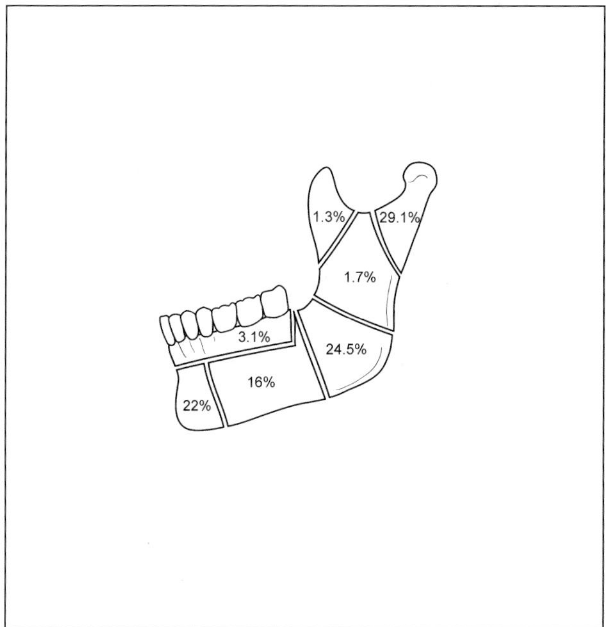

Figure 11–3 Incidence of mandibular fractures by region.

Symptoms and Physical Findings

- Pain
- Malocclusion–document the angle class of occlusion
- Trismus – inability to completely open mouth due to pain
- Crepitus/bony step-offs
- Mandibular instability
- Edema and ecchymoses over fracture site
- Contusions, lacerations, and excoriation
- Intraoral
    - Dental hygiene (abscesses?)
    - Buccal or lingual ecchymosis
    - Avulsed teeth/loose teeth
        - Use the numbering system to account for avulsed, loose, fractured, or missing teeth
    - Lacerations
- Open bite
- Deviation of jaw on opening – suggestive of condylar fracture
- Paresthesia/anesthesia – document function of inferior alveolar, lingual, and mental nerves
- Transection of the inferior alveolar nerve can result in paresthesia/anesthesia at the lips, teeth, and gums
- Assess TMJ with finger in external auditory canal – condylar head should translate anteriorly without significant pain if joint is not injured

Radiographic Evaluation

A Panorex radiograph **(Fig. 11–4A)** offers the best diagnostic tool in suspected mandible fractures. It is a quick and inexpensive radiograph that offers a complete view of the mandible. It provides an easy means of identification of symphyseal and angle fractures, as well as showing the relation of the fracture line to teeth. Some minimally displaced fractures at the symphysis may be difficult to visualize on a Panorex. Patients are required, however, to have their C-spines cleared because the Panorex radiograph is taken in the sitting position. Otherwise, an intubated or obtunded patient can undergo a panoramic zonography or Zonarc (a panoramic evaluation in the supine position).

CT evaluation is cost effective and offers a near 100% sensitivity for diagnosing mandibular fractures (**Figs. 11–4B, C**). A CT of the face with coronal reconstructions should be ordered for patients who demonstrate a high index of suspicion for a mandible fracture. Each CT should also be complemented with a Panorex radiograph to show the relation of the fracture line in relation to the mandibular teeth. This detailed information on dental occlusion in relation to the fracture is not easily seen on CT and is important when assessing which teeth may need to be extracted to allow for optimal mandibular union. Coronal CT evaluation is also helpful in diagnosing mandibular coronoid and condyle fractures (**Fig. 11–4B**).

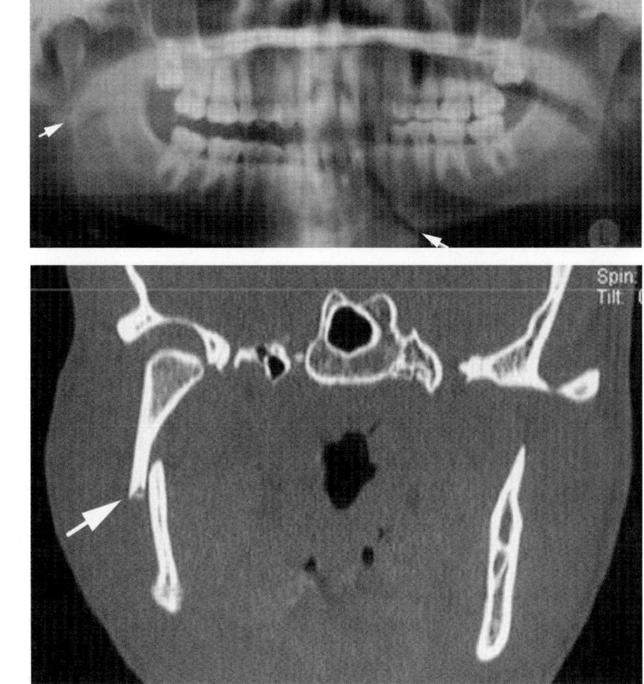

Figure 11–4 Mandibular fractures of the symphysis commonly occur in combination with fractures of the contralateral condylar region. **(A)** Panorex radiograph clearly illustrating the fracture of the parasymphysis. **(B)** CT coronal scan pf the same patient demonstrating a subcondylar fracture not easily seen on the Panorex radiograph.

(Continued)

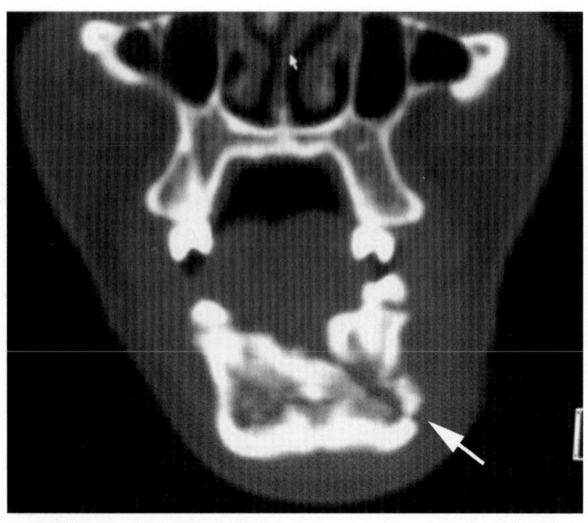

C

Figure 11–4 *(Continued)* **(C)** Evaluation of the parasymphyseal fracture by coronal CT.

Classification of Fracture

Types of Fracture

- Closed versus open
- Displaced versus nondisplaced
- Complete versus incomplete
- Linear versus comminuted
- Favorable–when the muscles draw the bony fragments together
- Unfavorable–when the fragments are displaced by the forces of the muscles.

Location of Fracture (Fig. 11–1)

- Symphyseal – between central incisors
- Parasymphyseal – between distal border of canine and central incisor
- Body – between distal edge of canine and distal border of third molar
- Angle
- Ramus

- Coronoid
- Condyle
  - Condylar head
  - Condylar neck

Nonoperative Management

The absolute goal in the treatment of mandibular fractures is establishment of preinjury occlusion. Additionally, attention should be placed on reestablishment of facial contour, height, symmetry, and projection. These goals are accomplished by achieving anatomical reduction of the fracture fragments without infection and with normal mandibular motion.

Immobilization techniques depend on the degree of displacement and the fracture location. Nonoperative management is instituted when the fractures are single, nondisplaced, and patients exhibit preinjury occlusion.

Criterion for Nonoperative Treatment of Mandibular Fractures	Indications for Operative Treatment of Mandibular Fractures
Isolated to one region	Fractures of multiple regions
Nondisplaced	Displaced
Simple	Comminuted
Patient exhibits preinjury occlusion	Poor occlusion
	Failed Nonoperative management
	Associated Infection

These patients are counseled to comply with a nonchew diet and to perform aggressive oral hygiene for 6 weeks. Nonoperative candidates treated conservatively should be monitored closely at 1- or 2-week intervals until fracture healing. During this observation period patients should be evaluated for maintenance of occlusion and signs of infection. Deviation of a normal prognosis may portend operative management.

- Discharge to home
  - Nonchew diet for 6 weeks

- Good oral hygiene – tooth brushing and Peridex (3M, St. Paul, MN) mouthwash swish-and-spit every 2 to 4 hours
- Follow-up in clinic within 2 weeks, obtain additional Panorex radiographs, and assess occlusion

Surgical Treatment

Generally, surgical treatment for mandibular fractures is recommended for patients with comminuted, displaced, infected, or multiple injuries. Treatment strategies in the acute setting include bridle wiring and closed reduction in maxillomandibular fixation (MMF) with arc bars and wires or elastics (**Fig. 11–5**).

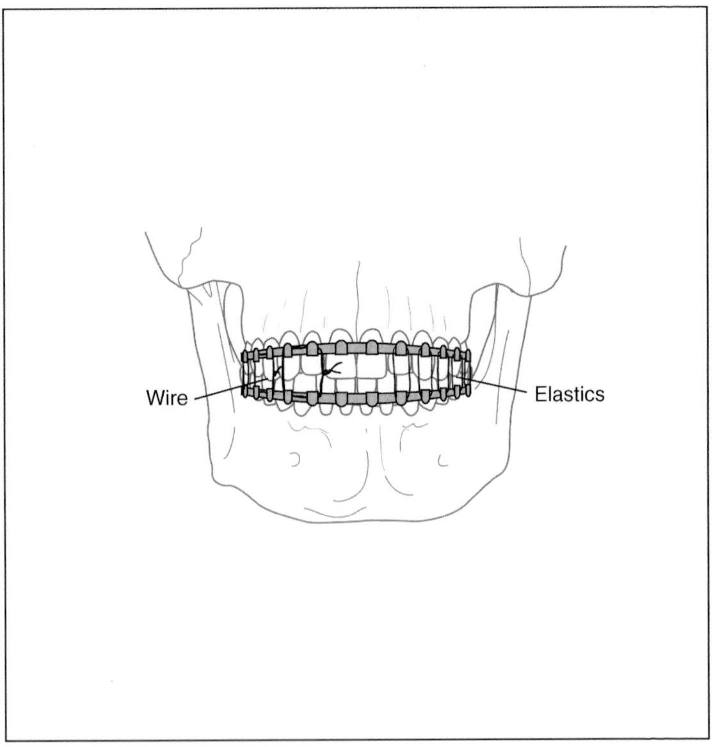

Figure 11–5 Closed reduction of mandible fractures utilizing arch bars with elastics or wire fixation.

The specific fracture management depends on the region. Once operative treatment has been decided, reduction of the fragments should be undertaken to reduce the possibility of infection, pain, and malunion. If fracture reduction is to be delayed more than 5 days, the fracture fragments should be stabilized with Barton bandages (see Chapter 7, Fig. 7–5), a cervical collar externally or alternatively with MMF until surgery. Fixation of open fractures should be attempted within 72 hours.

For patients admitted for operative treatment:

- Prophylactic antibiotics – clindamycin 600 mg IV q6h
- Ensure patient airway. Patients with mandibular fractures may have tongue-based airway obstruction (lacerations etc.) that may require tracheostomy
- Rule out C-spine injuries
- Clear liquid or nonchew diet
- Oral hygiene – tooth brushing and Peridex mouthwash swish and spit every 2 to 4 hours
- IVFs
- Preoperative workup

Condylar Fractures

Condylar fractures are treated conservatively with closed reduction or open reduction depending on the degree of displacement and laterality. Treatment strategies in this region are employed to decrease the incidence of ankylosis of the TMJ. Closed reduction is advocated in children or when the fracture pattern is high and contained within the capsule. Open reduction and internal fixation (ORIF) is advocated when there is significant displacement outside the capsule of the TMJ or into the middle cranial fossa. Foreign bodies within the capsule and failed closed reduction are additional indications for open reduction and internal fixation.

Unilateral nondisplaced fractures in patients with normal occlusion can be treated conservatively. Patients are placed on a nonchew diet and encouraged to perform rehabilitation protocols to prevent ankylosis.

Displaced unilateral fractures in patients with malocclusion are treated with closed reduction for 7 to 10 days, after which rehabilitation is begun.

Bilateral nondisplaced fractures in a patient with a stable midface are treated with closed reduction. However, bilateral displaced fractures or bilateral fractures in a patient with an unstable midface should be considered for ORIF of at least one side to preserve mandibular height and ensure occlusion.

Coronoid and Ramus Fractures

Coronoid fractures, if isolated are managed conservatively provided the patient can open and close the mouth normally. Those patients unable to range normally or with significant pain should undergo ORIF. When coronoid fractures occur in combination with other mandible fractures, ORIF of the concomitant fracture is recommended over closed reduction to prevent ankylosis.

Due to the splinting mechanism of the insertion of the muscles of mastication on the ramus, these fractures are stable unless severely displaced. Ramus fractures in isolation are treated with closed reduction.

Angle Fractures

The angle of the mandible is the thinnest portion of the bone and is additionally weakened by the presence of the third molar. Fractures in this region commonly occur secondary to direct trauma and in isolation. The angle lacks dentition and incurs significant distracting forces from the masseter and the temporalis negating the ability for closed reduction to establish occlusion. Therefore, angle fractures are treated with ORIF.

Body and Symphyseal Fractures

Due to the presence of dentition in this region, fractures of the body and symphysis are treated with closed reduction if they are single and easily reducible. If significant dentition is missing or the fracture pattern is comminuted or irreducible, ORIF is considered.

Fractures in this region of the mandible commonly occur with contralateral fracture to the subcondylar area. Therefore, careful examination of the condyles is warranted in these patients.

Severely Comminuted Fractures

These fractures are associated with severe bony distinction as well as possible soft tissue loss. These fractures may require external fixation and débridement in the operating room. Establishment of an airway and ruling out C-spine injury are of paramount importance.

12

Examination of Hand Injuries

♦ History

1. Determine the patient's
   - Age
   - Sex
   - Hand dominance
   - Occupation
   - Other medical problems
2. Confirm
   - Location of the injury
   - Cause of the injury
   - Time of the injury
   - Duration of the injury process

♦ Physical Examination

First, perform a general exam of the hand:

- Verify any physical hand deformities
- Establish if there is any bleeding, pain, swelling, recent deformity, and ecchymosis
  - Can herald a closed fracture
- Confirm open wounds
- Note old scars
- Assess posture of the hand

    - Angulation of digits signals possible dislocations and fractures
- Palpate fingers, palm, and wrist for tenderness
- Determine the temperature of the hands and if they are dry or moist

Patient complaints of severe pain, paresthesia, and swelling of the hand, may indicate flexor tenosynovitis. These symptoms can be explained by Kanavel signs.

Kanavel Signs
• Pain over tendon sheath • Fusiform swelling of digit • Finger held in flexion • Pain on passive extension (Hallmark sign)

Range of Motion

Check the resting hand position; this may indicate tendon injuries if the natural arcade is disrupted. Ask the patient to move all joints of the hand. Look at movement holistically and at each individual joint's movement. Start with the fingertips and move proximally. **Table 12–1** lists the normal ROM for each joint in the hand.

Distal Interphalangeal Joint

Look for tuft fractures distal to this joint. Normal ROM is 0-degree extension and 65 degrees of flexion. Also, look for Mallet finger, which is a result of the avulsion of the terminal extensor tendon, leaving the DIP joint in a flexed position. Stabilize the middle phalanx with the PIP joint extended to test flexion of the flexor digitorum profundus (FDP).

Table 12–1 Normal Range of Motion for Joints of the Hand

Joint	Degrees of Flexion
Finger DIP	65
PIP	110
MCP	85
Thumb IP	90
MCP	45–60

Proximal Interphalangeal Joint

Look for full ROM from 110 degrees of flexion to zero degrees extension in this joint. Inability to flex the PIP joint can result from disruption of the flexor digitorum superficialis (FDS) tendon/muscle, volar plate disruption, or contracture of the intrinsic muscle of the hand. Inability to extend the joint may be a result of extensor mechanism injury (boutonniére deformity) or contracture of the flexor mechanism.

Metacarpophalangeal Joint

The digit MCP joints progress through 85 degrees of flexion and zero degrees of extension. Often, tendons or the joint capsule may be exposed in cases of laceration. In cases of assault, look for an open laceration over the joint along with decreased prominence of the fifth metacarpal head. This signals the possibility of the fracture of the fifth metacarpal neck (boxer's fracture). Joint dislocations may also be present. These may be difficult to reduce if tendons or volar plate entrapment occurs.

The Thumb

Normal MCP joint ROM for the thumb is 45 to 60 degrees of flexion and zero degrees of extension. Look for radial and ulnar deviation and pain in the MCP and CML joints. Radial deviation at the MCP joint is a sign of weakness of the ulnar collateral ligament (gamekeeper's thumb).

Common Hand Deformities

Boutonniére Deformity

- PIP flexion with DIP extension caused by disruption of the extensor insertion of middle phalanx and volar migration of the lateral bands

Swan Neck Deformity

- PIP hyperextension with DIP flexion caused by lateral band tightness and volar plate laxity

Table 12–2 Intrinsic and Extrinsic Flexors and Extensors of the Hand by Joint

Joint	Flexion	Extension
Finger DIP	FDP	Lumbricales, interossei
Finger PIP	FDP, FDS, FDM, FPB	EDC, lumbricales, interossei
MCP	Lumbricales, interossei	EDC, EIP, EDM, EPB
Thumb IP	FPL	EPL
Wrist	FCR, FCU, PL	ECU, ECRL, ECRB

Abbreviations: FDP, flexor digitorum profundus; FDS, flexor digitorum superficialis; FDM, flexor digiti minimi, FPB, flexor pollicis brevis; EDC, extensor digitorum communis; FPL, flexor pollicis longus; EIP, extensor indicis proprius; EDM, extensor digiti minimi; EPB, extensor pollicis brevis; EPL, extensor pollicis longus; FCR, flexor carpi radialis; FCU, flexor carpi ulnaris; PL, palmaris longus; ECU, extensor carpi ulnaris; ECRL, extensor carpi radialis longus; ECRB, extensor carpi radialis brevis.

Extrinsic Muscles of the Hand (Table 12–2)

Flexors

Each of the extrinsic flexors is responsible for flexion across one or more joints. Care must be taken to isolate and test each of these tendons individually. The flexors can be injured at their muscle bellies in the forearm or their tendinous portions in the hand. The flexors of the digits include the FDP, FDS, and the flexor pollicis longus (FPL). The wrist is flexed by the combination of the flexor carpi ulnaris (FCU) and flexor carpi radialis (FCR) muscles and secondarily with extension of the finger flexors.

Testing

FDP Hold the patient's PIP joint in extension and ask the patient to flex the DIP joint. The FDP can flex both joints if one is not immobilized (**Fig. 12–1**).

FDS Hold all fingers in full (PIP and DIP) extension except the one digit whose FDS tendon you are testing. Ask the patient to flex his or her finger. If the FDS is uninjured, then the PIP will flex. The muscle bellies of the FDS tendon can work independent of each other when the FDP tendons are pulled together. Therefore, immobilize all of the digits in extension so the FDS tendon can be tested of each digit (**Fig. 12–2**). The only exception to this rule is the FDP of the index finger. To

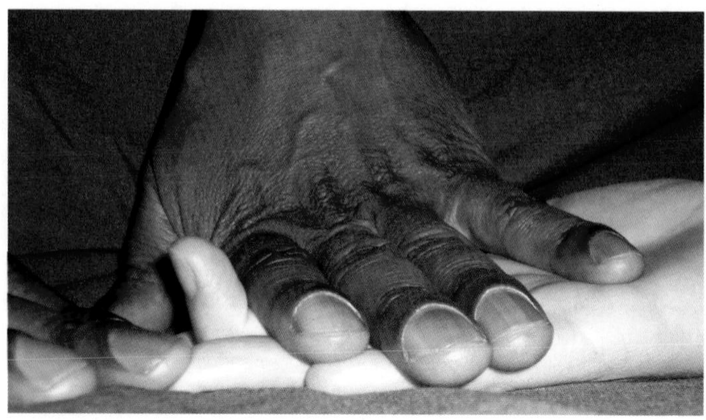

Figure 12–1 Physical examination of flexor digitorum profundus (FDP). Isolate the FDP by immobilizing the PIP joint, thereby minimizing the contribution of the FDS tendon.

determine if the FDS is intact in the index finger, have the patient hold a sheet of paper between the thumb and index finger. If the PIP joint in the index finger is flexed (due to the presence of FDS) then the FDS is intact. If the PIP joint is extended, then the FDS is not intact. Fifteen percent of the general population do not have small finger FDS; it is not functional in another 15%.

FPL Ask the patient to flex his or her thumb IP joint.

Extensors

The extrinsic extensors can be damaged at their muscle bellies in the dorsal forearm all the way to the distal phalanx. They are grouped into six compartments. The MCP joint is extended by the extrinsic extensors only while the PIP and DIP joints are extended by the combination of the intrinsic and extrinsic extensors. The compartments and tests of the extrinsic extensors are as follows:

Compartment 1 Abductor pollicis longus (APL; abducts thumb) and extensor pollicis brevis (EPB; extends MCP joint)

- APL: Abduction of thumb on flat surface (**Fig. 12–3**)
- EPB: Extension of thumb MCP joint

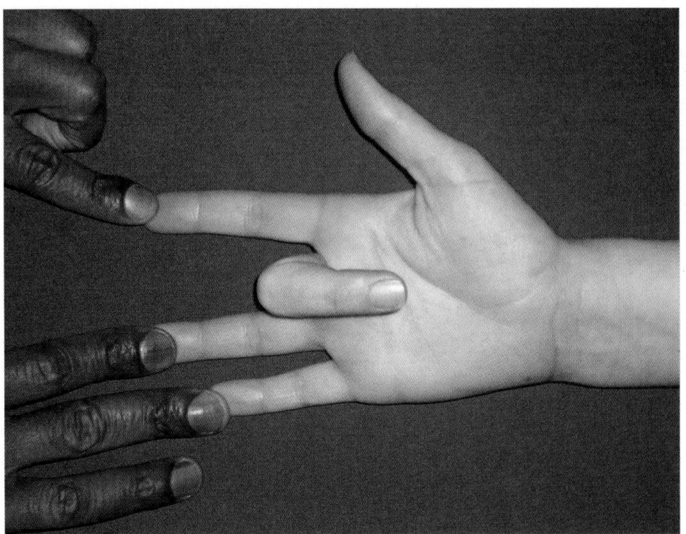

Figure 12–2 Physical examination of the flexor digitorum superfiscialis (FDS). Immobilize other digits in extension to minimize contribution of FDP to finger flexion.

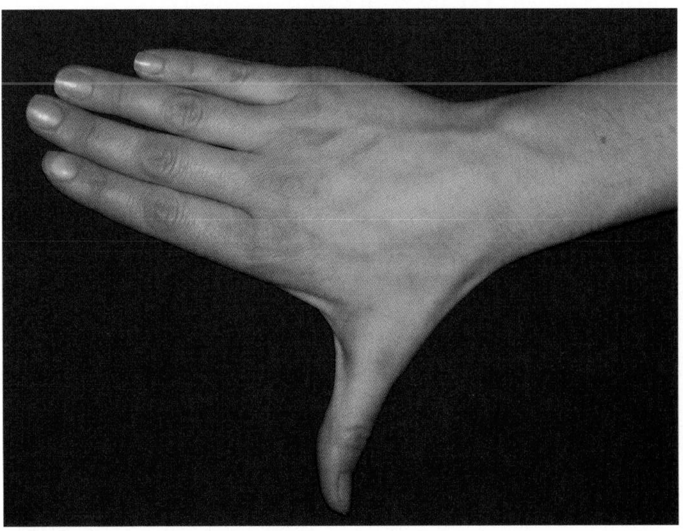

Figure 12–3 Physical examination of abductor pollicis longus (APL) and extensor pollicis brevis.

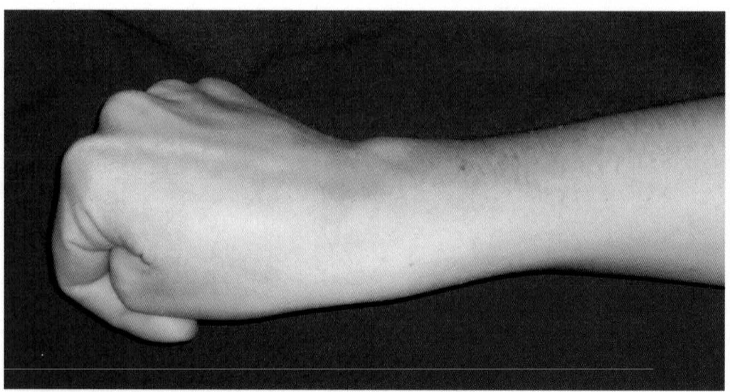

Figure 12–4 Finkelsten's test. See text for details.

- Finkelstein's test: Tests for de Quervain tenosynovitis. Have the patient make a fist over thumb and deviate hand ulnarly. This reproduces patient's pain (**Fig. 12–4**).

Compartment 2 Extensor carpi radialis longus and brevis, extend wrist

- Make a fist and extend wrist against resistance

Compartment 3 Extensor pollicis longus

- Put hand on a table and raise thumb off the table (**Fig. 12–5**)

Compartment 4 Extensor digitorum communis (EDC) and extensor indicis proprius (EIP)

- EDC: Extend all fingers

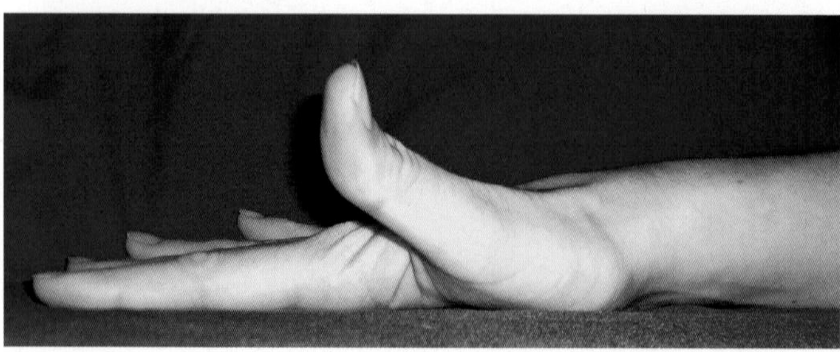

Figure 12–5 Physical examination of extensor pollicis longus.

- EIP: Ask patient to hold index finger in extension while flexing other fingers. EDC tendons are grouped and therefore cannot act independent of each other.

Compartment 5 Extensor digiti minimi

- Hold small finger in extension while making a fist with other fingers

Compartment 6 Extensor carpi ulnaris

- Extend the wrist ulnarly and palpate tendon over fifth metacarpal

Intrinsic Muscles of the Hand (Table 12–2)

The muscle bellies and tendons of these muscles are contained within the hand. Together these muscle act to flex the MCP joint while extending the IP joints. The intrinsic muscles of the hand are listed below, together with the appropriate tests.

Thenar muscles Abductor pollicis brevis, opponens pollicis, flexor pollicis brevis

- Palpate thenar eminences. If hypotrophic, consider median nerve damage. To test these muscles, ask the patient to perform thumb pulp to small finger pulp opposition.

Adductor pollicis Involved in pinching

Hypothenar muscles Abductor digiti minimi, flexor digiti minimi, and opponens digiti minimi

- Palpate hypothenar eminence. Ask the patient to abduct small finger.

Interosseous muscles MCP flexion and IP extension

- Dorsal: Digital Abduction
- Palmar: Digital Adduction
    - Hold IP joints in extension and ask the patient to flex the MCP joint

Lumbricales muscles MCP flexion and IP extension

- Hold MCP in flexion and ask patient to extend IP joints

♦ Vascular Examination

Look to see if the hand is cold, congested, or edematous. Check capillary refill by pinching fingertips and counting the time it takes to refill; 2–3 seconds is normal. Check for blue or necrotic spots on the fingertips.

Palpate radial and ulnar arteries. If not palpable, then use Doppler ultrasound. Perform Allen test to determine the integrity of the palmar arch. First, ask the patient to make a fist while you occlude the radial and ulnar artery. Then have the patient open the exsanguinated hand. Let go of the radial vessel and determine if the hand returns to its normal pink hue. Repeat this procedure and let go of the ulnar artery. If the patient cannot make a fist, then use a Doppler to find the palmar arch. Occlude the radial or ulnar artery and check to see if there is a Doppler signal in the palmar arch. Perform test on both radial and ulnar artery. Make sure to examine the arch throughout its course in the palm. Next, examine each of the digital arteries using the same technique as described above.

♦ Neurological Examination

The radial, ulnar, and median nerves supply the hand; **Table 12–3** gives distributions and innervation. First determine if the patient has sensation over the radial distribution (the back of the hand).

Table 12–3 Nerve and Motor Innervations of the Hand

Nerves	Motor	Sensory
Radial	Triceps Anconeus Brachioradialis Supinator Extensor carpi radialis brevis Extensor carpi radialis longus Extensor carpi ulnaris Extensor digitorum communis Extensor indicis proprius Extensor digiti minimi Abductor pollicis longus Extensor pollicis longus Extensor pollicis brevis	Dorsal wrist capsule Dorsal radial hand Dorsal thumb, index, middle, radial half of ring finger to PIP joint
Ulnar	Flexor carpi ulnaris Flexor digitorum profundus (small and ring fingers) Palmaris brevis	Ulnar half of the dorsum of hand Volar and dorsal aspect of small finger, ulnar side of

(Continued)

Table 12–3 *(Continued)*

Nerves	Motor	Sensory
	Dorsal interosseous muscles Palmar interosseous muscles Ring and small finger lumbricales Adductor pollicis Flexor pollicis brevis deep belly Hypothenar muscles: Abductor digiti minimi Flexor digiti minimi Opponens digiti minimi	ring finger
Median	Pronator teres Pronator quadratus Palmaris longus Flexor carpi radialis Flexor digitorum superficialis Flexor digitorum profundus (index and middle fingers) Flexor pollicis longus Index and middle finger lumbricales Thenar muscles Abductor pollicis brevis Opponens pollicis Superficial belly of flexor pollicis brevis	Volar wrist, thumb, index, middle finger and radial half of ring finger extending to the DIP joint

Next, turn the hand volar and determine if the patient has general sensation over the radial three digits and palm (median nerve). Make sure to examine the proximal portion of the palm for sensation. Finally, examine the volar and dorsal ulnar portion (ulnar nerve distribution).

To determine if digital nerves are intact perform the Weber test. Using a caliper or bent paper clip to measure the minimum distance of two-point discrimination. Normal is 2 to 3 mm in the finger pulp. Patients involved in occupations where heavy labor is required may have a two-point discrimination of 5 to 6 mm. Patients who are blind may have a discrimination of 1 to 2 mm. The patient needs to be correct in 7 tests out of 10 for good two-point discrimination.

Table 12–4 The Medical Research Council Muscle Grading System

Observation	Muscle Grade
No contraction	0
Flicker or trace of contraction	1
Active movement, with gravity eliminated	2
Active movement against gravity	3
Active movement against gravity and resistance	4
Normal power	5

Testing motor nerve function of the upper extremity is performed by eliciting contraction of specific motor units.

Musculocutaneous nerve Flexes the elbow

Radial nerve Stimulates elbow extension

Median nerve Wrist, finger (index, long), and thumb flexion

Ulnar nerve Wrist, finger (ring, small), and intrinsic hand motility including abduction and adduction of the fingers

Radial nerve Wrist, finger (MP joint), and thumb extension

Specific nerve–muscle associations are listed in **Table 12–3**. In assessing motor function, the Medical Research Council Muscle Scale is useful for quantifying strength (**Table 12–4**).

13

Anesthesia and Splinting of the Hand and Wrist

♦ Anesthesia

The application of nerve blocks not only provides comfort to patients, but it also assists the physician in exposing and repairing injuries to the upper extremity.

- Lidocaine 1 to 2%
  - Toxic dose >4 mg/kg
- Lidocaine 1% with epinephrine 1:100,000
  - Toxic dose >7 mg/kg
- Marcaine 0.25% (Abbott Laboratories, Abbott Park, IL)
  - Toxic dose >2.5 mg/kg
- 1:1 mixture of Lidocaine/Marcaine
  - Toxicity is the same for both agents.
  - Toxicity is not additive.

Injection of Local Anesthetics

- Dilute the concentration
  - Dilute with sterile injectable saline
    - Provides additional volume for injection over a larger area without increasing the total dose administered
    - Aids in decreasing the total dose required
- Administer the local anesthetic agent slowly

- Toxicity develops due to peak serum concentration
  - Inject each site sequentially rather that all at once
  - Spread the total dose of local anesthetic over a longer period; this leads to lower peak serum levels
- Add epinephrine
  - Effective concentrations 1:1,000,000
  - Improves safety and allows administration of lower doses
  - Improves hemostasis, thus decreasing duration of procedures
  - Helps prevent the need for subsequent injection
  - Beware of epinephrine in use in patients with cardiac history
  - Avoid administering epinephrine in the digits and to pediatric patients
- Add bicarbonate
  - Decreases burning on administration
  - Add 1 cc of a 1 mEq/mL bicarbonate for every 9 cc of local anesthesia
- Consider mixing agents
  - Use more than one local anesthetic to take advantage of the unique properties of each local anesthetic
  - Use a short-acting local anesthetic (lidocaine) with a long-acting (Marcaine)
  - Provides prolonged anesthesia without causing toxicity from either agent
  - The toxicity of the mixture does not exceed the individual toxicity of each agent.
  - Toxicity of multiple agents in a solution is not additive.
- Always draw back prior to injection to ensure no anesthetic is given intravascularly

Digital Nerve Block

Two volar and two dorsal nerves innervate the digit. The common digital nerve and dorsal sensory nerves are blocked via a dorsal approach with one needle stick. Using a 25-gauge needle, a 1-cc wheel is made over the extensor mechanism at the level of the MCP joint to block the dorsal sensory nerve. The needle is then advanced volarly on either side of the joint in the web space until it is palpated in the palm. An additional 1 cc of local anesthesia is placed on each side to block the digital nerve.

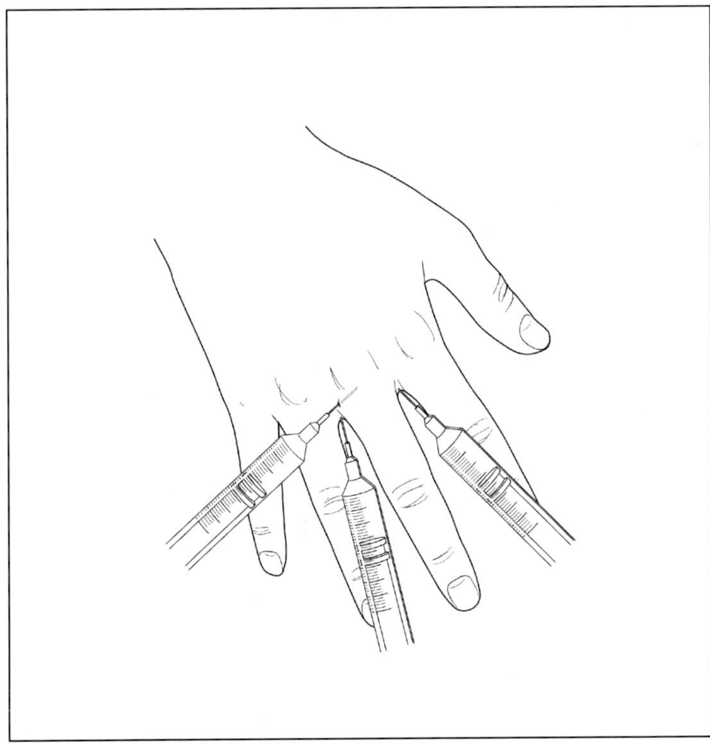

Figure 13–1 Digital nerve block.

Alternatively, a digital nerve block may be performed with direct instillation of the 1 to 3 cc of anesthetic agent in the adjacent web spaces dorsally and dorsal over the MCP joint (**Fig. 13–1**). Care must be taken not to perform circumferential instillation around the digit that may subsequently impair perfusion.

Wrist Block

Wrist blockade includes anesthesia of the median, ulnar, and radial nerves. The efficacy of a wrist block is increased by application of a tourniquet at the mid-forearm. Wrist blocks are applied as follows:

Median nerve Inject 5 cc agent between the palmaris longus and flexor carpi radialis tendons at the proximal wrist crease using a

25-gauge needle. Avoid injection directly into the median nerve. If the patient feels tingling during injection, withdraw the needle 1–2 mm and reinject.

Ulnar nerve Inject 5 cc of agent radial to the flexor carpi ulnaris tendon at the wrist crease with the wrist in flexion. We must take care not to inject into the ulnar artery. Remember to draw back on the syringe first.

Radial nerve – superficial branch Inject 5 cc of agent from the midpoint of the dorsum of the wrist to the radial border of the anatomical snuffbox (**Fig. 13–2**). Draw back on the syringe so as not to inject into the radial artery.

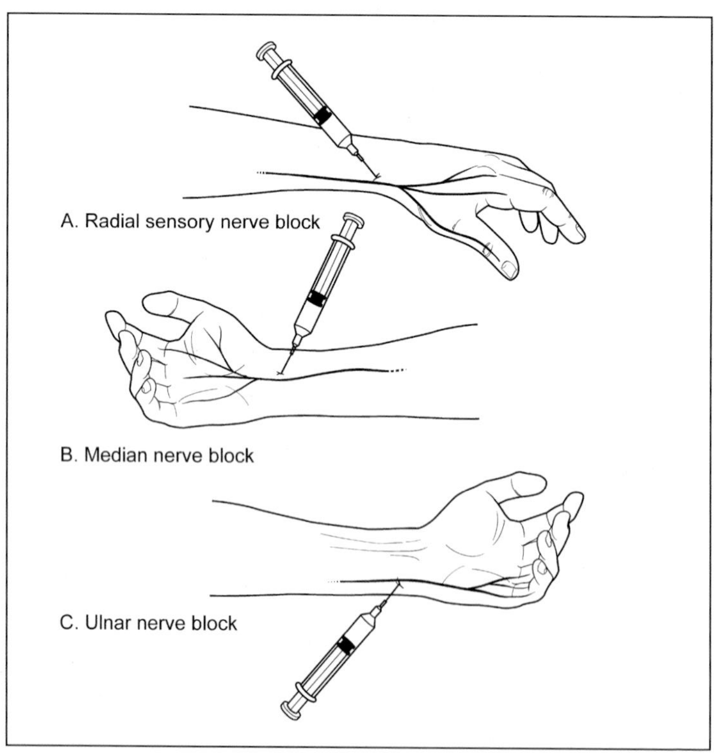

Figure 13–2 Wrist blocks. **(A)** Radial sensory nerve block. **(B)** Median nerve block. **(C)** Ulnar nerve block.

♦ Splinting

The proper splinting of fractures and dislocations is of paramount importance. The use of a splint in tendon, nerve, and arterial repair protects against traction and disruption of the repair. Splints of the hand for infections and soft tissue trauma prevent dysfunctional bone and soft tissue contractures. The use of a splint also helps to decrease a patient's pain and discomfort.

General Procedures (Fig. 13–3A)

- Use local and regional blocks to allow painless manipulation of the extremity while splinting

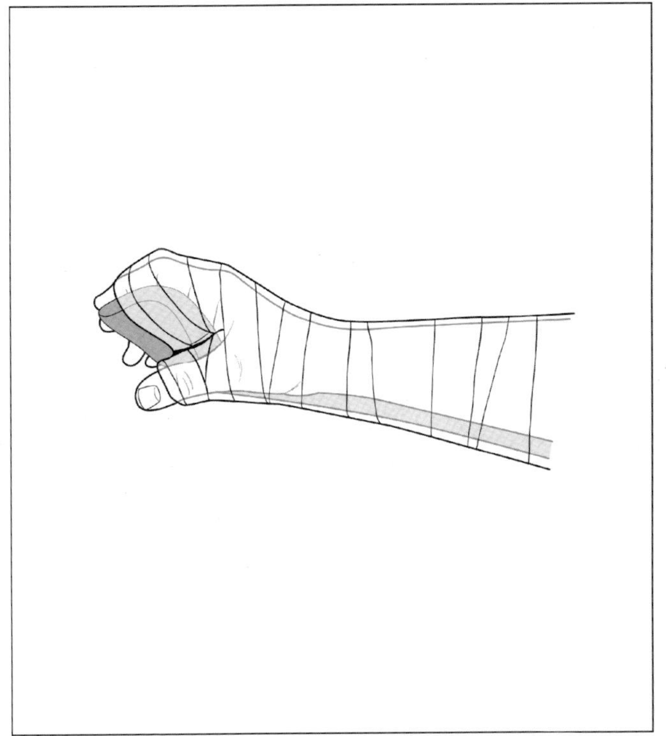

Figure 13–3A–H Volar splint. The gray shading denotes plaster position.

(Continued)

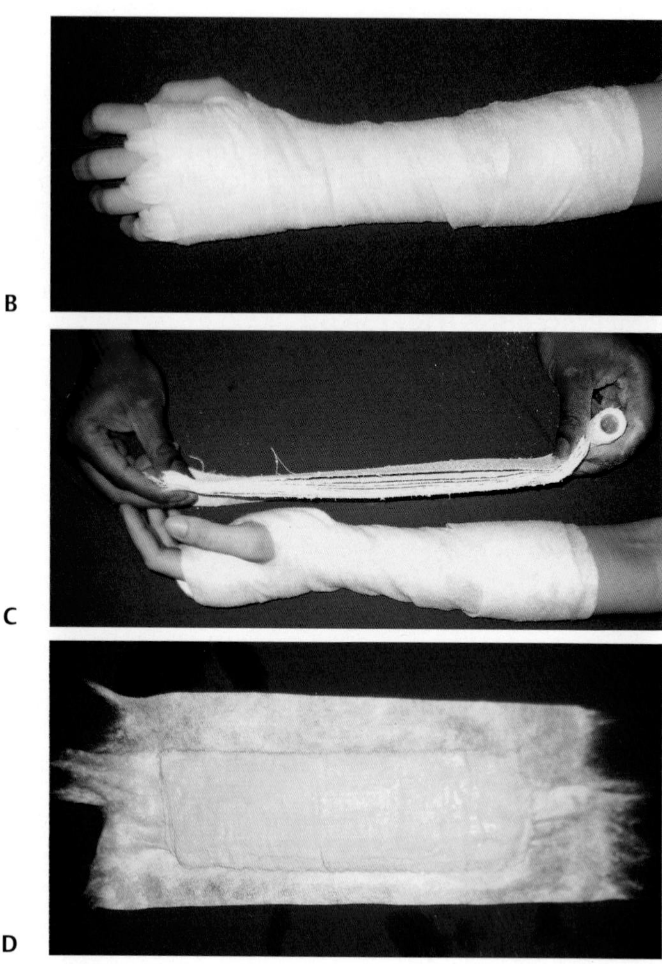

Figure 13–3B–H Placement of a plaster, step by step; and plaster in palce. See text for description.

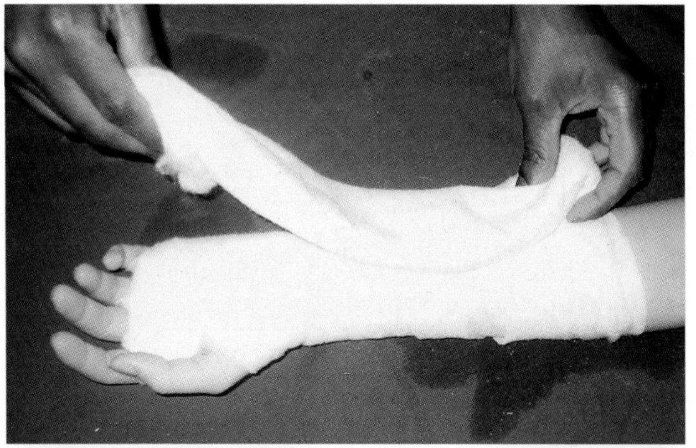

E

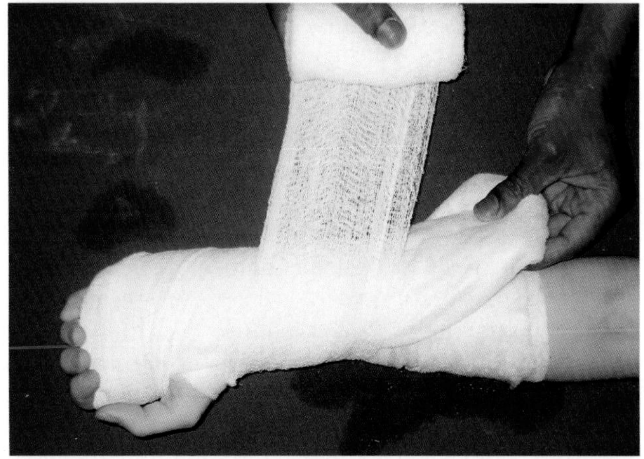

F

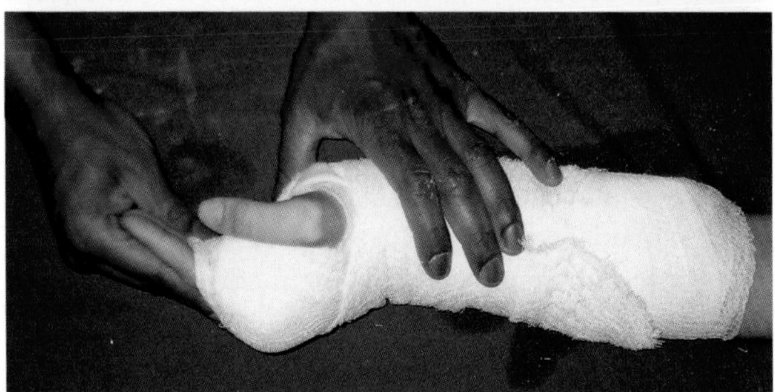

G

(Continued)

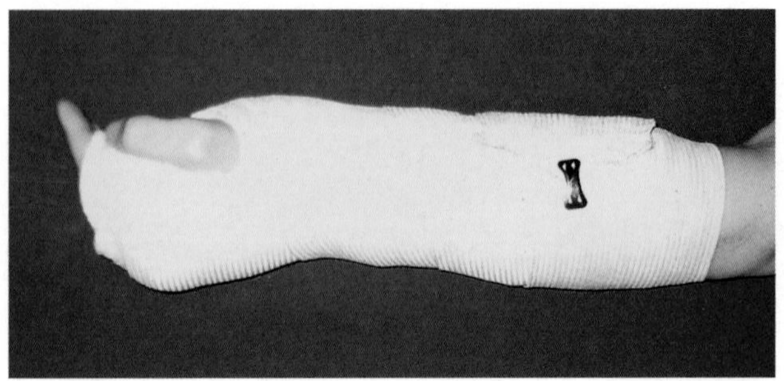

H

Figure 13–3B–H: (*Continued*)

- Splinting materials used are
  - Kerlix (Kendall Company, Mansfield, MA) gauze
  - 4-inch (10 cm) web roll
  - 4-inch plaster material
  - 4-inch Ace bandage
  - 4-inch coband
- After injury repair, clean and dry the extremity
- Place a single layer of Webril (Kendall Company, Mansfield, MA) around the hand and forearm loosely
- Measure the length of the area to be splinted; cut a 10-ply piece of plaster material at that length. Alternatively, premade plaster/gauze of fiberglass composites (e.g., OCL) can be cut to length and used.
- Wet the plaster material and place it on the hand/forearm in the desired position
- Place plaster in Webril wrap (**Fig 13–3D**)
- Hold the plaster material in position by wrapping with a single layer of Kerlix
- Apply either Ace or coband in a single loose layer over the splint
- Apply circumferential wraps *loosely* to avoid constriction
- Elevate the extremity to prevent dependent edema while in the splint
- Prescribe a short-term follow-up protocol especially in outpatient treatment, to allow assessment for edema digital perfusion and splint displacement

Splint Types

*Volar Splint (**Fig. 13–3**)*

- Most versatile splint for radial-sided injuries
- Index and long finger fractures
- Index and long finger infections
- Wrist neurovascular injuries
- Forearm infections
- Metacarpal fractures

Position (intrinsic plus position)

- Proximal forearm to DIP joint
- Apply on volar surface of the forearm/wrist and hand
- Include index through small finger
- Keep thumb free
- Extend wrist 35 degrees
- Flex MCP joint 90 degrees
- Flex PIP/DIP joints 0 to 10 degrees
- For extensor tendon injuries, place MCP joint in extension.

*Ulnar Gutter Splint (**Fig. 13–4**)*

- Ulnar-sided injuries
- Ring and small finger fractures
- Ring and small finger infections
- Extensor tendon injuries
- Ulnar-sided metacarpal fractures

Position

- Proximal forearm to DIP joint
- Apply on ulnar volar surface of the forearm/wrist and on the hand to the mid-dorsum
- Include ring and small fingers
- Keep thumb, index and long finger free
- Wrist extended 35 degrees
- Flex MCP joint 90 degrees
- Flex PIP/DIP joints 0 to 10 degrees

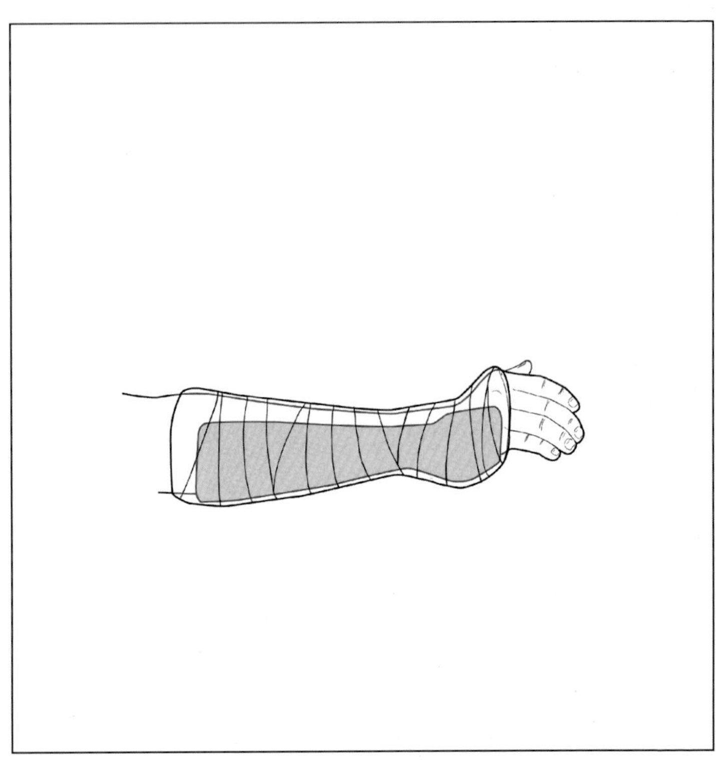

Figure 13–4 Ulnar gutter splint. The gray shading denotes plaster position.

*Thumb Spica Splint (**Fig. 13–5**)*

- Most versatile splint for thumb injuries
- Thumb fractures and dislocations
- Thumb and thenar infections
- Thumb tendon injuries
- Scaphoid injuries
- First metacarpal fractures

Position

- Proximal forearm to IP joint
- Apply two plaster splints
  - One on volar surface of the forearm/wrist and thumb
  - One radially to the mid-dorsum

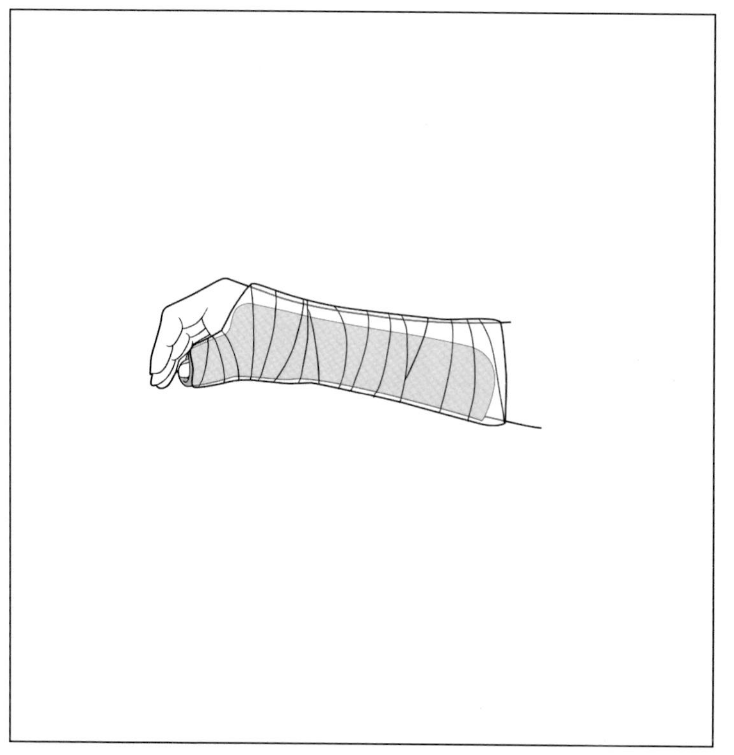

Figure 13–5 Thumb spica splint. The gray shading denotes plaster position.

- Keep index through small finger
- Extend wrist 35 degrees
- Scaphoid injuries
- Flex MCP joint 10 to 15 degrees
- Flex IP joint 0 to 10 degrees

*Extension Block Splint (**Fig. 13–6**)*

- Flexor tendon injuries
- Proximal and middle phalangeal fracturs (**Fig. 13–7**)

Position

- Splint from proximal forearm to DIP joint
- Apply on dorsal surface of the forearm/wrist and hand

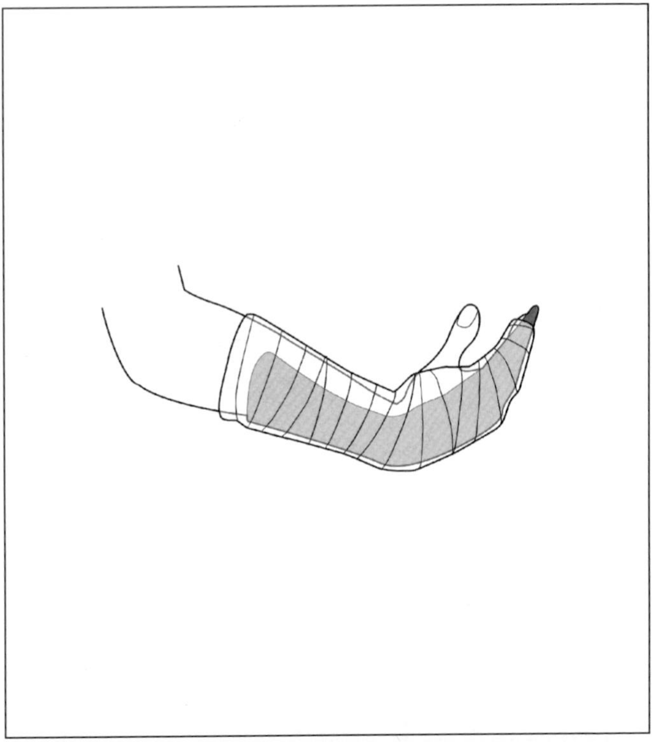

A

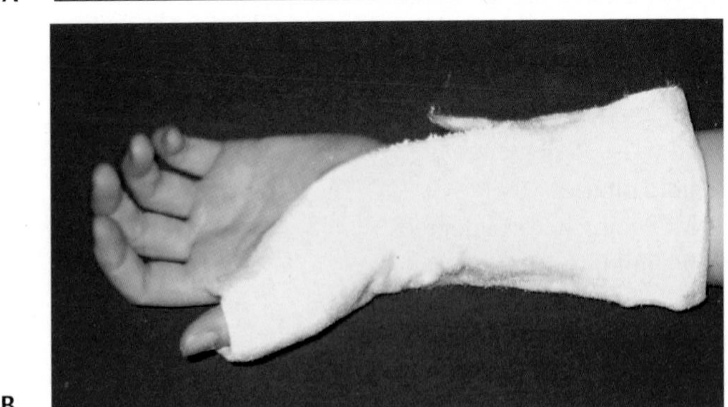

B

Figure 13–6A, B Extension block splint. The gray shading denotes plaster position.

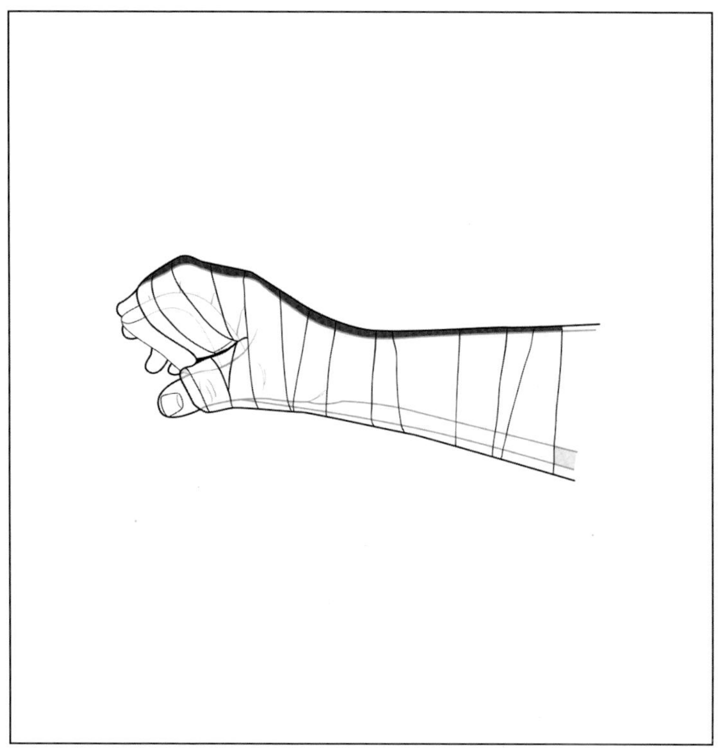

Figure 13-7 Dorsal extension block splint in intrinsic plus.

- Include index through small finger
- Flex wrist 45 degrees
- Flex MCP joint 90 degrees
- Flex PIP joint 45 degrees
- Flex DIP joint 20 degrees
  - Splint from proximal forearm to DIP joint
  - Apply on dorsal surface of forearm
  - Include adjacent finger and digits
    - Wrist in neutral or slight extension
    - MP in 70–90° flexion
    - IPs extended

14

Hand and Wrist Fractures and Dislocations

♦ The Hand

Physical Examination

A complete physical examination to determine the integrity of the neurovascular, musculoskeletal, and cutaneus system is warranted. Dedicated hand series radiographs should include AP, true lateral, and oblique views. In selected cases of carpal fractures and wrist injuries, a CT scan may be indicated.

Fracture Classification

- Open versus closed
- Displaced versus nondisplaced
- Transverse versus oblique versus spiral versus comminuted or avulsion
- Traumatic versus pathologic
- Adult versus pediatric
  - In pediatric patient: Green stick versus epiphyseal plate
  - In epiphyseal plate: Salter-Harris classification

Fracture Treatment

In general, hand fractures can be treated in the emergency room with closed reduction and splinting. However, if the fracture is open, displaced, unstable, or if the angulation is not acceptable, then operative treatment may become necessary.

Open Fractures

- Perform a finger or wrist block
- Culture and irrigate open fractures profusely
- Administer IV antibiotics (ER treatment or inpatient)
  - Ampicillin 500 g IV q8h + gentamycin 3 to 5 mg/kg q.d. divided 8 hours (check peak and through serologic levels)
  - Vancomycin 1 gm IV q12h + Ceftriaxone 1 to 2 gm IV q24h
  - Outpatient prophylactic antibiotic for patients with plan for later surgery includes Bacitracin DS and PO b.i.d.
- Irrigate the wound and splint the patient in preparation for operative reduction

Phalangeal and Metacarpal Fractures

Indications for Operative Treatment

- Intraarticular fracture
- Irreducible fractures
- Malrotation
- Subcapital phalangeal fractures
- Open fracture if displaced or angled
- Bone loss
- Multiple fractures
- Fractures with soft-tissue injury

Phalangeal Fractures

Distal Phalanx Fractures

Distal phalanx fractures are the most common fractures in the hand. The thumb and middle finger are most likely involved. Patients present with tuft fractures, shaft fractures, and intraarticular injuries due to crush.

Tuft Fractures

Open Fractures

- Perform finger or wrist block
- Remove nail

- Irrigate
- Repair nail bed with 6.0 to 7.0 chromic and stent the nail matrix (see Chapter 17, Fig. 17–2)
- Immobilize DIP joint in extension with tongue blade or aluminum splint for 3–4 weeks with PIP free
- In cases of severe comminution, soft-tissue repair is adequate for splinting fractures
- Treat with Bacitracin DS and PO b.i.d. × 5 days

Closed Fractures

- Perform finger or wrist block
- If a hematoma is present under the nail, drain it with a drill (sterile 18-gauge needle tip), heated paper clip, or electrocautery
  - If the hematoma >50% of nail bed, likely nail bed injury
    - Remove and repair nail bed and splint with piece of foil from chromic package or use the nail itself (see Chapter 17, Fig. 17–2)
      - Splint finger for 2 weeks
      - Treat with outpatient antibiotics × 5 days

Shaft Fractures

- Nondisplaced
  - Repair soft tissue
  - Splint 3 weeks
  - Bacitracin DS and P. O. b.i.d.
- Displaced
  - Likely nail bed laceration
  - Repair nail matrix (see Chapter 17, Fig. 17–2)
  - Stabilize fracture with K-wire or 18-gauge needle
  - Splint finger with PIP free for 3 weeks
  - Outpatient antibiotics × 5 days

Intraarticular Fractures

- Open fracture
  - Repair nail bed

- Splint DIPJ in extension for 6–8 weeks
- Outpatient antibiotics
- Closed fracture
  - Splint DIPJ in extension

Dorsal Base
An intraarticular fracture of the dorsal base (mallet fracture) is a hyperflexion injury in which a portion of the dorsal bone breaks off with extensor mechanism. It causes extensor lag with a mallet finger deformity. Treatment requires strict patient compliance. In pediatric population this may require a K-wire through DIPJ.

- Treat with splint in extension for 6 to 8 weeks

Volar Base (FDP Avulsion)
An intraarticular fracture of the volar base is a hyperextension injury in which the flexor digitorum profundus (FDP) pulls off the distal phalanx.

- Treat with ORIF because FDP may retract into palm
- Splint hand in emergency room with tongue blade or aluminum splint
- If open, wash out, repair nail bed, start antibiotics, and splint

Middle and Proximal Phalanx Fractures

Middle and proximal phalanx fractures are caused by crushing forces rather than direct blow, twisting, or angular forces. If these fractures are nondisplaced or stable, simply buddy tape or splint with IP extended for 3–4 weeks. A comminuted, displaced fracture of the middle or proximal phalanx proximal to the articular surface is called a pilon fracture.

Articular fractures

- In ER setting
  - Fracture of single digit: ensure involved joint is in extension
    - Aluminum or tongue blade splint
  - Multiple fractures: Splint hand in intrinsic plus
  - Follow up in clinic for operative management

- Non-displaced: Inherently unstable.
  - Operative management using either closed or open reduction and fixation by multiple k-wires or screws or a combination.
  - If non-operative management chosen then close follow up required
- Displaced
  - Dorsal base fractures of middle phalanx
    - ORIF to avoid Boutonniers defect
  - Dorsal base fractures of proximal phalanx
    - Requires ORIF
- Unicondylar (Displaced)
  - Inherently unstable either closed or open reduction and fixation with multiple K-wires or screws
  - Extension splint 2-3 weeks
- Bicondylar
  - Requires ORIF
  - Non-comminuted
    - Fix condyle to condyle first then to the shaft with K-wires or screws
  - Comminuted
    - Difficult to treat
    - DIPJ:
      - Minimal displacement: Closed reduction.
        - Splint 2 weeks in extension
        - Physical therapy in 2 weeks
      - Displaced:
        - ORIF with K-wire/screw fixation
        - Early motion at 2 weeks
    - PIPJ:
      - Skeletal traction of the middle phalanx for 3–4 weeks with forearm splint.
      - Active flexion of PIPJ immediately

Nonarticular fractures

- Shaft
  - Non-displaced and stable- **not *rotated, angulated, or comminuted***

    - Splint the finger in extension with an aluminum splint
        - Must cover proximal and distal joint
        - Duration of 1 week
        - Once pain and swelling resolve then buddy tape to adjacent finger and begin range of motion
- Displaced but amenable to stable closed reduction
    - Usually ***transverse*** fractures not oblique or spiral
    - Attempt reduction and stabilization
        - Perform digit block (See Chapter 13, Fig. 13–1)
        - Flex MPJ maximally
        - Flex distal fragment to correct volar angulation
        - Dorsal splint in intrinsic plus position
            - Plaster should be placed dorsally for extension blocking. MP 90°, IP extended, include adjacent digits in splint for stabilization
        - Splint for 3 weeks, then buddy tape for additional 2 weeks
- Unstable—if potential for rotation or angulation exists
    - Open, oblique, spiral, comminuted fractures
    - Radiographically angulated
    - Assess by having patient flex finger
        - Fingers overlap
        - Plan closed reduction with percutanous pinning with in 3-4 days
        - Use 0.035-0.045 inch
    - Unstable transverse fractures
        - Intramedullary longitudinal fixation through metacarpal head with k-wire
        - Extension block splint in intrinsic plus position with IP joints free for 3-4 weeks
    - Comminuted fractures
        - Require operative management
        - External fixation device often indicated
            - Preserves length
            - Assists with management of soft tissue injuries
    - For unsuccessful percutaneus pinning perform ORIF with plates or interaosseous wireing

Base fractures of proximal phalanx

- Extraarticular
  - Angulation of 25° in adults and 30° in children requires treatment
  - To reduce:
    - Flex MP maximally
    - Flex distal fragment to correct volar angulation
  - Splint in intrinsic plus (dorsal plaster) for 3 weeks
  - Failed closed reduction
    - K-wire fixation

Metacarpal Fractures

Head Fractures

- Open fractures 2° to closed-fist injury (fight bite)
  - Wrist or local block
  - High-pressure irrigation and débridement
  - Leave wound open
  - Delay fixation until sign of fixation subsided
  - Splint in intrinsic plus volar splint (See Chapter 13, Fig. 13–3)
  - Augmentin 875 mg P. O. b.i.d. × 10 days
  - Short-term follow-up
- Index finger most commonly involved due to axial loading and often intraarticular
- AP, lateral, and oblique x-rays; if not clear, then Brewerton view
- Nondisplaced: Splint in volar splint for 4 weeks (see Chapter 13, Fig. 13–3)
  - If >25% of articular surface or >1 mm step-off → splint in safe position, plan ORIF
  - Mini-plate fixation preferred, to allow early mobilization (Fig. 13–3)
- If comminuted, perform wrist block and wash out wounds
  - Splint acutely in safe position
  - Plan for immobilization for 2 weeks with skeletal traction, external fixation, or arthroplasty

Neck Fractures

- Reduction indicated
  - Pseudoclawing (clawing of fingers with ulnar nerve intact)
  - MCP hyperextion/PIP flexion
  - Rotational deformity
  - Scissoring of fingers
  - Unacceptable angulation

Apex dorsal angulation occurs from intrinsic muscle contraction.

Treatment based on angulation:

- Small digit (Boxer's fracture) – 50 degrees angulation acceptable
- Ring finger – 30–40 degrees angulation acceptable
- Middle and index finger – 10 to 15 degrees acceptable

If angulation is unacceptable, and pseudoclawing or rotation deformity present:

- In fresh fracture attemp closed reduction
- In fracture > 7 days old then may require operative reduction
- Closed reduction by Jahss maneuver: First perform a wrist block (wrist block for boxer's fracture)
- Next, flex MCP joint to 90 degrees and PIP joint to 90 degrees
- Apply upward pressure on the proximal phalanx while pressing down on the metacarpal shaft (**Fig. 14–1**)
  - If reduced, splint in safe position for 3 to 4 weeks and monitor reduction regularly (Fig. 13–3) for 2nd-3rd metacarpal
  - For 4th, 5th metacarpal fracture use ulnar gutter splint (See Chapter 13, Fig. 13–4)
  - If not reducible, use internal fixation with K-wires, plates, or dorsal tension band wires
    - Splint in a safe position acutely
  - After reduction take radiograph to confirm reduction

Shaft

The types are

Spiral: Torsional forces with 5 degrees of malrotation causing a 1.5-cm digital overlap

Oblique: Lateral bending forces with axial load

Transverse: Lateral bending force versus axial load

Comminuted: Direct impact on the metacarpal, which may cause shortening

If angulation is acceptable (see above Neck Fractures section), then close reduce the fracture using traction and a wrist block.

- Flex MP joint
- Press on the fracture apex dorsally with a palmar directed force
- Place in volar intrinsic plus splint

If there are multiple fractures, the fracture is unstable/open, or there is scissoring and severe angulation, then ORIF with K-wires, interosseous wires, plates, lag screws, or external fixation. In the emergency room, place the patient in a safe-position splint.

Base Fractures/CMC Joint Fracture–Dislocation

These are inherently unstable fractures caused by axial load versus direct blow. Index finger and middle fingers are less likely to undergo this type of fracture because these joints are less mobile. Hamate-fifth metacarpal intraarticular fracture is a Baby (reverse) Bennett fracture.

- Because the extensor carpi ulnaris pulls on the fifth metacarpal, in the x-rays you will see that the ulnar portion subluxes proximally and dorsally.
- Closed reduction with K-wires versus ORIF. In the emergency room, place the patient in a volar splint in safe position (see Chapter 13, Fig. 13–3)

Thumb Fractures

Injuries occur by direct trauma and angular or rotary forces.

Phalangeal Fractures

Extraarticular:

- Proximal phalanx fracture with $> 20–30°$ apex volar angulation is unacceptable and requires reduction

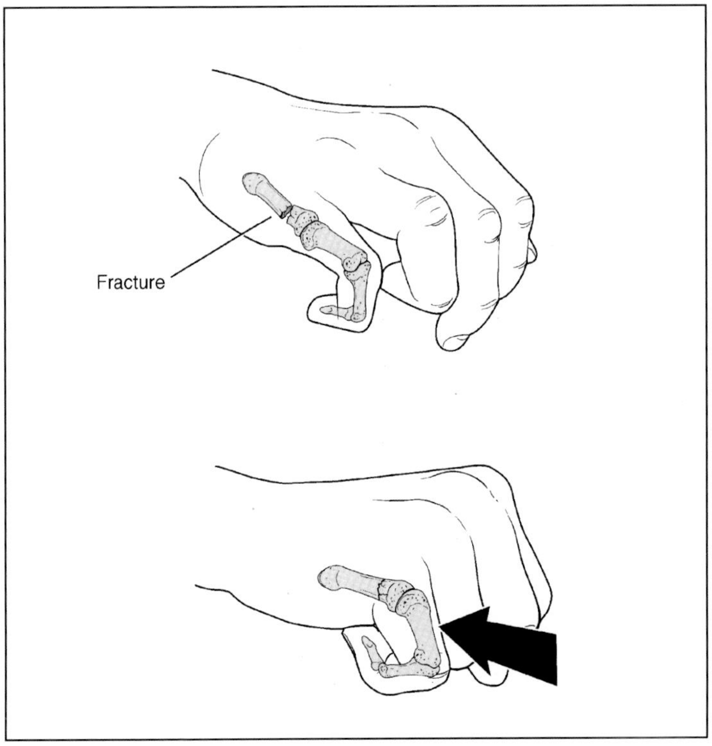

Figure 14–1 Jahss maneuver for reduction of metacarpal fractures.

- Distal tuft: Associated with subungual hematoma, nail bed injuries, and comminuted fractures
  - Finger block
  - Remove nail
  - Irrigate thoroughly
  - Repair nail bed
  - Splint 3 to 4 weeks in extension with tongue blade or aluminum splint
- Transverse shaft
  - Finger or wrist block
  - Close reduce
  - Splint in extension, if unstable then ORIF

Intraarticular: Occurs when axial load is placed on partially flexed thumb

- Dorsal base avulsion = mallet thumb
  - Treat with 6–8 weeks of extension splint
  - Consider ORIF if subluxation present
- Volar base fracture
  - Consider avulsion of flexion pollicis longus
- Fractures of the ulnar base represent avulsion of the ulnar collateral ligament and represent "skier's thumb" or "gamekeeper's thumb"
- If fragment is displaced >2 mm or > 25% of articular surface, then K-wire fixation versus ORIF
- In the emergency room, place in a thumb spica splint (See Chapter 13, Fig. 13–5)

Metacarpal Fractures

Head and shaft fractures result from torsional, direct impact, angulatory, or rotary forces.

Extraarticular:

- Fractures up to 30° angulation are acceptable due to compensation by CMC mobility.
- Head: Rare fracture that requires reduction and K-wire fixation versus ORIF if displaced. Can attempt closed reduction by Jahss maneuver (**Fig. 14–1**).
- Shaft: After radial and median nerve block at the wrist close reduce and splint in thumb spica splint (Fig. 13–5)

Intraarticular:

- Bennett fracture: Occurs when partially flexed thumb is axially loaded.
  - It is defined as intraarticular fracture–subluxation of the base of the first metacarpal. On X-rays, the volar ulnar aspect of the metacarpal base remains stable due to the anterior oblique ligament. However, the rest of the metacarpal moves dorsally, proximally, and radially due to the pull from the abductor pollicis longus.

- If the bone fragment is >20% of CMC joint surface then close reduce and pin
  - If the fracture cannot be reduced in a closed fashion, then ORIF
  - In the emergency room, splint in a thumb spica splint and plan operative treatment (Fig. 13–5)
- Rolando fracture: Any comminuted intraarticular fracture of the base of the first metacarpal, but traditionally referred to as Y- or T-shaped intraarticular fractures
  - If severely comminuted, use skeletal traction and perform percutaneous fixation
  - If fracture contains large fragments, only ORIF
  - In emergency room place in thumb spica splint (Fig. 13–5) and plan operative treatment

Pediatric Phalangeal and Metacarpal Fractures

Children rarely present with fractures of the hand. When they do, the chance of displacement is less than in adults. This is due to the malleability of the child's bones as well as the tougher periosteum. Fractures are classified into either nonepiphyseal (66%) fractures or fractures that involve the epiphysis. Epiphysis fractures are categorized by Salter-Harris classification (**Fig. 14–2**). Fractures in children heal twice as fast as in adults and the epiphyseal plate compensates for angular deformity of the fractures. However, accurate reduction is crucial in intraarticular fractures.

Extraarticular Fractures

Fractures commonly occur in the middle and proximal phalanx in children.

- If the fracture is not displaced (type I), splint in a safe position
- If decreased (type II) or no (type III) bone contact between the fragment and remainder of the bone, then use K-wire fixation
- In the emergency room, splint the hand in a safe position (See Chapter 13, Fig. 13–2)
- In infants, may have to include the elbow in flexion along with dorsally placed plaster.

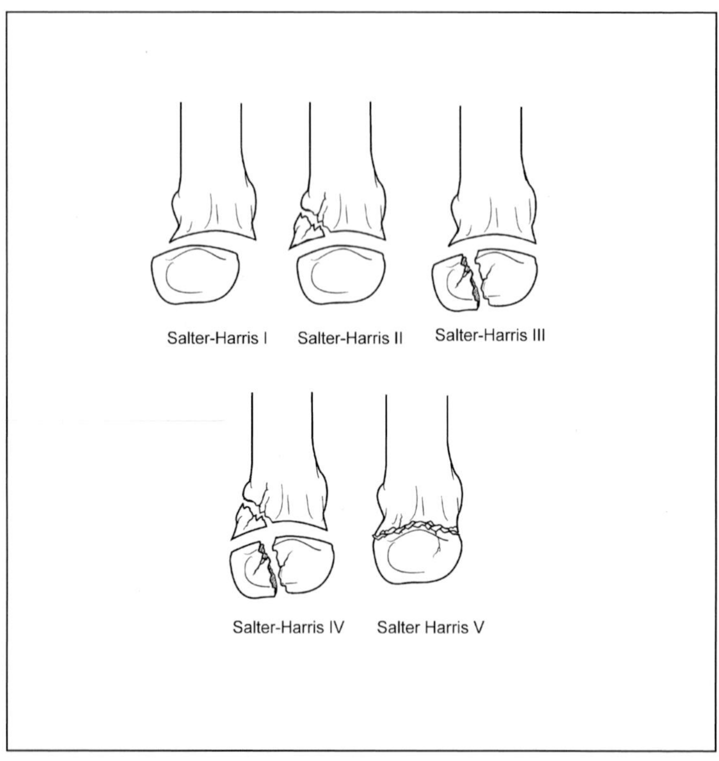

Figure 14–2 Salter-Harris classification of epiphyseal fractures.

Intraarticular Fractures

- In cases of displaced fractures, ORIF with miniaturized wires (0.028–0.039 in) and screws – especially in children >2 years old

Epiphyseal Fractures (Fig. 14–2)

Salter-Harris I A fracture through the epiphyseal plate with separation of epiphysis from the metaphysis (shear injury). This usually occurs in early childhood when the plate is thick with a zone of hypertrophying chondrocytes and sparse calcification. The prognosis is good with wrist block, reduction, and splinting the hand in a safe position (See Chapter 13, Fig. 13–2). May require dorsal plaster in young children.

Salter-Harris II This fracture involves a metaphyseal fragment associated with an epiphyseal fracture. This is the most common Salter-Harris fracture. The prognosis is good with adequate reduction.

Salter-Harris III This fracture occurs in children >10 years of age due to avulsion force. It is an intraarticular fracture through the epiphysis, and the epiphyseal plate. Unless accurate reduction is performed, the prognosis is poor.

Salter-Harris IV This is a rare fracture that occurs at any age. The fracture extends from the articular surface through the epiphysis, through the epiphyseal plate, and involves a portion of the metaphysis. It has a poor prognosis unless an accurate reduction performed.

Salter-Harris V This is an extremely rare fracture that occurs at any age. It is caused by crushing of the epiphyseal plate by axial load. It has a poor prognosis due to growth arrest.

♦ Dislocations

Phalanx and Metacarpal Dislocations

Proximal Interphalangeal Joint

The PIP joint is stabilized by a combination of thick collateral ligaments, accessory collateral ligaments, and the volar plate. This is a hinge joint with an arc of rotation of 100 to 110 degrees and is the most common site of ligamentous injury. The direction of dislocation is dependent on the position of middle phalanx at the moment of joint dislocation.

Types of Dislocation

Volar: Rare, caused by rotary longitudinal compression force on a semiflexed middle phalanx

Dorsal: Result of longitudinal compression and hyperextension

Stability

Active: Ask patient to move through full ROM. If subluxation occurs, the patient has severe ligamentous injury. If the patient has full ROM without subluxation, then adequate stability exists.

Passive: Hold finger in full extension and then at 30 degrees of flexion. Test lateral stress on the collateral ligaments. Compare stability to unaffected PIP joint.

Grades

Mild Joint stable with microscopic tears

Moderate Joint with abnormal laxity with moderate degree of tear

Complete Collateral ligaments are completely torn.

Treatment

Sprains

- Splint joint in extension for 2 to 3 days (with aluminum splint)
  - If it remains stable, start early motion

Dislocations

- Volar: Examine finger for the integrity of the central slip. After giving finger block, then reduce using traction and splint 2 to 3 days in extension (aluminum splint or tongue blade). If stable start early motion.
- Dorsal: If dislocation is stable after reduction, then splint in extension for 3 weeks. If dislocation is unstable after reduction, then surgery is required. These dislocations often involve >40% of the volar articular surface. Plan ORIF or volar plate arthroplasty.
- Lateral: Use a combination of buddy taping and extension splinting for 3 weeks. In nearly all cases, the ligaments return to their normal position even though they may have been completely disrupted.

Distal Interphalangeal Joint and Thumb Interphalageal Joint

Because both flexor and extensors insert on the distal phalanx and help stabilize the joint, this dislocation is rare. Dorsal and lateral dislocations with open wounds are most common.

- Perform a digital block (see Chapter 13, Fig. 13–1)
- Although these dislocations are rarely reducible, try to reduce it by using longitudinal traction and direct pressure on the dorsum of the distal phalanx; manipulate the distal phalanx into flexion
- Immobilize in a dorsal splint for 2 to 3 days with PIP joint free
- Then buddy tape and start conservative active motion

Finger Metacarpophalangeal Joint

The condyloid joint is usually dislocated in a dorsal or ulnar direction.

Dorsal: Most commonly occurs in index or small finger; caused by forced hyperextension
- ◦ Simple subluxation
- ◦ The volar plate usually stays with the proximal phalanx.

Treatment
Flex wrist to relax flexor tendons. Then flex the MCP joint by applying distal and volarly directed pressure to proximal phalanx. Do not apply traction or hyperextend as this will convert the injury to a complex dislocation.

- Complex dislocation: Volar plate is usually jammed into the joint; therefore, flexion and reduction are impossible.
  - ORIF and immobilize for 2 weeks
- Lateral: Radial collateral ligament is ruptured by the forced ulnar deviation while the MCP joint is flexed.
  - Reduce and immobilize in 30 degree of flexion for 3 weeks
  - Buddy tape with motion for 2 to 3 weeks
- Volar: This is extremely rare.
  - Attempt closed reduction
  - If reduction not stable, then ORIF

Thumb Metacarpophalangeal Joint

Gamekeeper's Thumb
Gamekeeper's thumb is the most common injury, which occurs when partially flexed thumb is axially loaded. This is defined as an avulsion-fracture from the ulnar base of the proximal phalanx due to disruption of ulnar collateral ligament. (See Chapter 13, Fig. 13–9).

Treatment
Immobilize joint for 6 weeks in thumb spica. Surgical exploration is indicated if joint continues to be unstable or if the ulnar collateral ligament is blocked by interposition of adductor pollicis muscle (Stener lesion).

♦ Wrist Injuries

The wrist is an anatomically complex structure that plays a vital role in all aspects of human life. The distal radioulnar (DRU) joint is a site at which hand supination and pronation occur as the radius rotates around the ulna. Distal to the DRU joint is the proximal carpal row, which is composed of the scaphoid, lunate, triquetrum, and pisiform. These bones articulate with the distal portion of the radius and ulna and allow for flexion and extension of the hand, as well as ulnar and radial deviation. Distal to the proximal row of carpal bones, is the distal carpal row, which is composed of the trapezium, trapezoid, capitate, and hamate. The distal carpal row and the second and third metacarpals form the "fixed unit" of the hand.

A detailed history that includes patient's occupation, hand dominance, detailed characterization of the mechanism of injury, as well as the location and level of pain should be the first step of evaluation. Three patterns of wrist injury exist: the perilunate pattern, the axial pattern, and injury from localized force concentration.

Perilunate Injuries

The injuries occur in an arc emanating from the lunate. The bones involved include the scaphoid, triquetrum, and capitate. If any of these bones are fractured, then the others should be checked for a fracture.

Axial Pattern Injuries

These injuries result from anteroposterior compression forces. These forces, generally occurring from an explosion or crush injury, propagate either on the ulnar or radial side of the capitate.

Single Bone Fractures

These usually are the result of a concentrated localized force.

Carpal Bone Fractures

Scaphoid

Most common carpal bone fractures occur in the wrist. By articulating with the lunate proximally and the capitate distally, the scaphoid stabilizes the wrist. Upon disruption, the wrist becomes more susceptible to collapse.

Mechanism
Fall on outstretched hand

Diagnosis
The patient has tenderness in the anatomic snuffbox and radial wrist pain. Order x-rays in AP, pronation oblique, supination oblique, and lateral views. Additionally, CT scans are useful in establishing the vascularity and degree of displacement. A clenched fist position may improve view. Look for a radiolucent line radial to the scaphoid on an AP view. If the line is preserved then the scaphoid is intact. If scaphoid is fractured, the line is displaced or obliterated (navicular fat stripe sign). (**Fig. 14–3**)

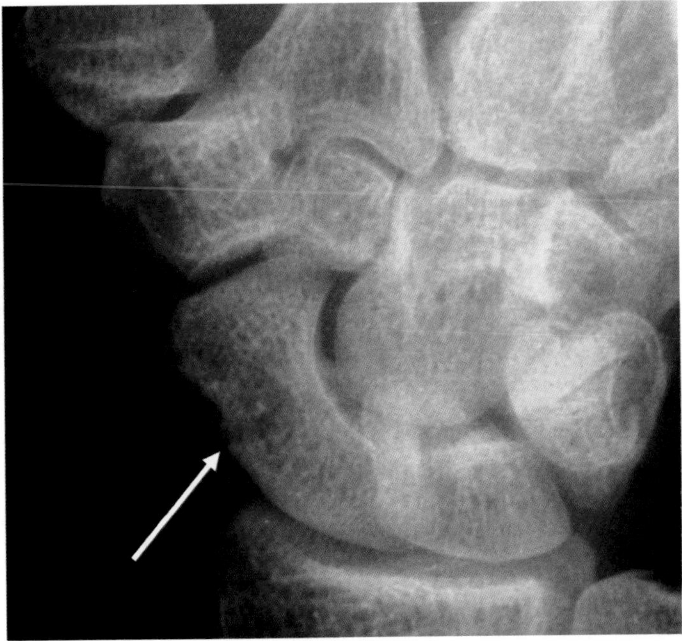

Figure 14–3 Fracture of the scaphoid.

Blood Supply

The superficial palmar branch and the dorsal carpal branch of the radial artery enter at the distal aspect of the scaphoid. A loss of blood supply due to fractures at the waist or the proximal portion of the scaphoid leads to avascular necrosis of the scaphoid (Preiser's disease) and future pain/instability.

Types of Fracture

- Horizontal oblique: Fracture of the scaphoid oblique to the longitudinal axis of scaphoid but perpendicular to the long axis of the limb (most common fracture of the scaphoid). Stable and usually treated with closed treatment in thumb spica for 6 to 8 weeks. (See Chapter 13, Fig. 13–5)
- Transverse: Scaphoid fractures that are perpendicular to the longitudinal axis of the scaphoid, but oblique to the limb. Less stable and less common than horizontal oblique fractures, these usually heal with 6 to 12 weeks of closed treatment (thumb spica). (Fig. 13–5)
- Vertical oblique: Rare and less stable; requires longer casting

Treatment

- Closed treatment: Reserved for suspected fractures and stable fractures with <1 mm displacement or a scapholunate angle <60 degrees or radiolunate fractures <15 degrees
- Place patient in thumb spica cast (Fig. 13–5) for 6 weeks (long arm cast and then 6 weeks in short arm cast).

Suspected Fractures

- Place the patient in thumb spica
- Technetium 99 methylene diphosphonate (Tc-99 MDP) bone scan in 2 weeks (time for bone at fracture site to resorb)
  - If negative, then no fracture exists
  - If positive, order a CT scan for determination of fracture site and further treatment

Nondisplaced Fractures

- Thumb spica cast until fracture heals (~ 6 weeks)
- Check for union

- Immobilize in a long arm cast for 6 weeks, then a short arm cast for an additional 6 weeks

Pediatric

- Rarely displaced; ORIF only in severe displacement
  - Otherwise, immobilize until skeletal maturity
- Surgical treatment
  - For open fractures of the wrist
  - Failed closed treatment (no healing in 12 weeks or nonunion after 6 months of casting)
  - Displacement >1 mm or scapholunate angle >60 degrees or radiolunate fracture >15 degrees
  - Very proximal fractures that are prone to avascular necrosis
  - If a patient has a nondisplaced fracture that cannot be immobilized, an arthroscopic approach can be taken.
    - Complications
      - Malunion
      - Avascular necrosis
      - Nonunion
      - Arthritis
      - Carpal instability
      - Scaphoid advance collapse

Other Carpal Bone Fractures

Mechanism
Fall on outstretched hand

Diagnosis
The patient has pain in the wrist; x-rays demonstrate fractures of carpal bones. If a fracture is suspected then the Tc-99 MDP will be positive in 2 weeks. A CT scan can also be performed for diagnosis of fractures, especially in the distal row. Triquetral fractures are caused by wrist hyperextension. Trapezial fractures are seen using the Betts view and often occur in cyclists.

Treatment

- Closed treatment
  - Nondisplaced carpal bone fractures should be immobilized for 6 weeks
  - Use a thumb spica for lunate fractures
  - Splint the hand in a safe position for capitate fractures
- Surgical treatment
  - Use for all open fractures and displaced fractures
    - Complications

Lunate Fracture

These may cause Kienbock's disease by affecting the lunate blood supply and causing avascular necrosis.

Hook of Hamate Fracture

These fractures are associated with racquet sports and golf; patients present with ulnar and volar wrist pain. The fracture occurs on impact with the ball. Nonunion is diagnosed with a CT scan. Removal of the Hook relieves the pain.

Pisiform Fracture

Nonunion is a common complication. Supinated oblique and carpal tunnel X-rays are most useful in diagnosing the fracture. Pain on nonunion resolves with removal of the pisiforms.

Scaphocapitate Syndrome

Scaphocapitate syndrome results from fractures in both the scaphoid and capitate wrist along with rotation of the capitate fragment 90 to 180 degrees. Treat with ORIF early. If missed, then treat expectantly. If symptoms persist, perform a wrist arthrodesis.

♦ Dislocations of the Wrist

Dislocations of the wrist range from perilunate ligamentous injuries to lesser arc injuries (dislocations only) to greater arc injuries (dislocation + fracture).

Scapholunate Ligamentous Injuries

As the force causing perilunate ligamentous injury increases, there is a predictable pattern of injury. The progression proceeds from scapholunate sprains to scapholunate dislocation, perilunate dislocation, and finally dislocation of the lunate. In severe cases, patients present with extreme dorsiflexion of the wrist.

Diagnosis

- Watson shift test: Put thumb on distal pole of scaphoid. Next, move joint radially, ulnarly, into extension and flexion.
  - Assess for pain or subluxation, which may herald instability
- Take stress radiographs
  - Scapholunate disruption

  On the AP x-ray, a scapholunate disruption can be seen between the scaphoid and lunate >3 to 4 mm (Terry Thomas/Letterman/Gap sign), or as a wedge-shaped lunate (piece of pie sign). If the lunate is rotated dorsally, then the patient has a dorsal intercalated segment instability (DISI) deformity. A volar dislocation of the lunate will be apparent as the spilled cup sign on lateral view (not associated with scapholunate disruption).

Treatment

If patient presents within 3 to 4 weeks of injury, then attempt closed reduction, which usually requires K-wire for fixation. If patient cannot be taken to surgery, then one can attempt closed reduction in the emergency room. This must be preceded by a thorough neurovascular examination. A hematoma block or brachial block can be performed.

Perilunate Dislocation
Initially, dorsiflex wrist and then slowly volar flex the wrist while holding the position of the lunate with the thumb of your other hand. Rearticulate the capitate and the lunate using pronation. Use fluoroscopy if needed.

Lunate Dislocation (Fig. 14–4)
Start with the procedure for perilunate reduction, then stabilize the lunate with your thumb and bring capitate into palmar flexion.

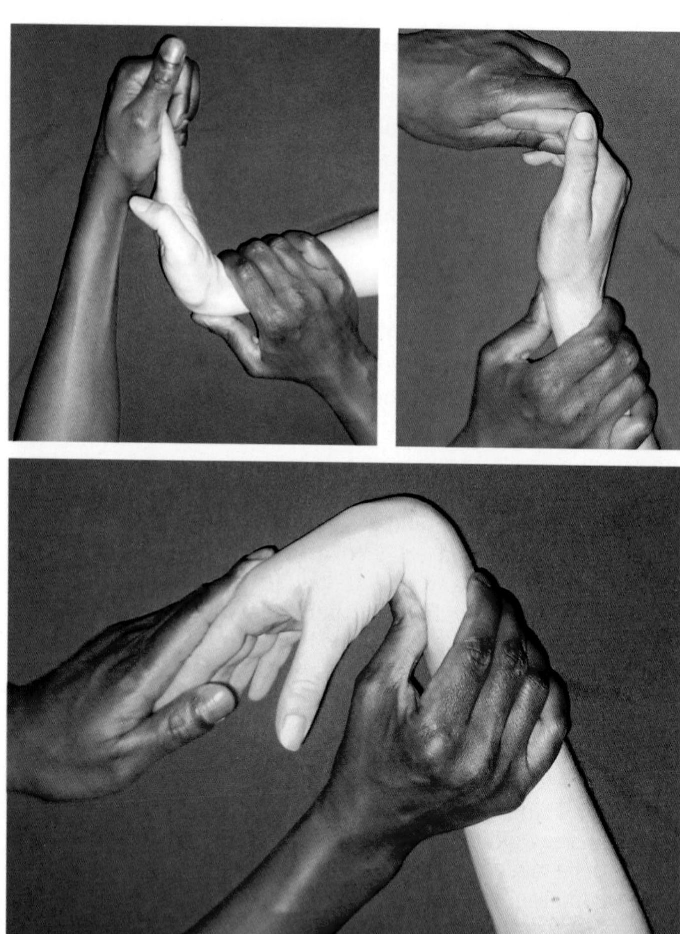

Figure 14–4 Reduction of a dislocated lunate. See text for details.

Scapholunate Dislocation

First dorsiflex the wrist and then radially deviate the wrist. If reduction is performed in the operating room (preferred), then K-wire the reduction. If reduction is performed in the emergency department, then attempt to place the patient in a splint in a thumb spica. If reduction does not hold, then you must perform ORIF.

Fracture Dislocations of the Wrist (Major Arc Injury)

The most common type is the trans-scaphoid perilunate fracture-dislocation. Use X-rays taken in traction for diagnosis. Usually requires ORIF.

Ulnar-Sided Ligamentous Injuries

The patient presents with tenderness on ulnar side of wrist (over lunotriquetral ligament) with possible avulsion fractures of the triquetrolunate ligament.

Diagnosis

- Ballottement test (Reagan Test)
  - Displacement of the triquetrum dorsally and volarly on the lunate with painful crepitus
- Lichtman test
  - Subluxation and pain with axial loading and deviation of wrist ulnarly
- X-ray
  - AP view demonstrates volar-intercalated segment instability (VISI) with volar-flexed scaphoid. Lunate is volar-flexed and triangular.

Treatment

Immobilize for 6 weeks in short arm cast

Triangular Fibrocartilage Complex (TFCC) Tears

The TFCC is a ligamentous and cartilaginous structure, which stabilizes the distal radioulnar joint and is the articulating surface for the ulnar carpus.

Diagnosis

- When patient grasps an object, wrist pain that worsens
- X-ray
  - Ulnar positive variance on X-ray
  - Arthroscopy versus MRI

Treatment

- Short arm cast for 6 weeks
- May do arthroscopy and débride of tears

15

Hand Infections and Injection Injuries

♦ Hand Infections

Hand infections are classified as superficial, deep, acute, subacute, or chronic. Ascertaining the cause of the infection, anatomical location, and length of duration of symptoms is essential to the proper diagnosis and the treatment of hand infections.

Hand infections range from superficial cellulitis to osteomyelitis. Cellulitis is a superficial inflammation of the dermal/epidermal components of the skin secondary to bacterial contamination. Deep to the dermis, infection in the subcutaneous tissue manifests as an abscess. Continual deep infectious penetration will affect the fascia or the synovial sheaths of the flexor and extensor tendons, particularly in the hand and forearm. These deeper infections warrant rapid evaluation and treatment to prevent necrotizing inflammation within the deep tissue planes and erosive extension into the hand and forearm.

Physical Examination

Patients with hand infections should receive a complete evaluation that begins with a physical examination. Key components include

- Inspection and palpation to determine location and to assess the depth of the infection
    - Remove all jewelry (watches, rings, etc.) to prevent secondary vascular constriction from a tourniquet effect when edema develops

- Assessment of neurovascular status
- Passive ROM assessment of all joints
- Obtain radiographs of the involved hand/digit – three views

Management

The antimicrobial treatments for common hand infections are described in **Table 15–1**. The antimicrobial therapies delineated in Table 15–1 represent empiric recommendations until definitive culture results are available for specific therapy.

Types of Hand Infections

Acute Paronychia

Acute paronychia is an infection that involves the eponychial, paronychial fold, or the nail matrix. This process usually begins under the skin of the lateral nail fold causing erythema and edema (paronychia). Persistent disease may cause extension into the eponychium (eponychia) or under the nail sulcus to the contralateral fold (runaround infection or horseshoe infection).

Etiology

- Poor fingernail hygiene
- Minor trauma
- Nail biting
- Finger sucking
- Manicures
- Artificial nails
- Hangnails

Treatment

An early infection without evidence of fluctuance can be treated conservatively:

- Warm soaks three times a day with a 1:1 solution of 3% hydrogen peroxide and normal saline
- Oral antibiotics for one week; consider anaerobic coverage (clindamycin 450 mg PO q.i.d.) for associated nail biting or finger-sucking etiologies (human bite)

Table 15–1 Antimicrobial Treatments for Common Hand Infections (Adult Doses)

Infection Type	Organism	Antimicrobial Therapy	Alternative Therapy
Cellulitis	Gram-positive cocci *Staphylococcus aureus* *Streptococcus*	Keflex 500 mg PO q6h **MRSA** Bactrim DS I PO b.i.d. or Clindamycin 450 mg PO q.i.d. or Vancomycin 1 mg IV q12h	**Penicillin allergic** Clindamycin 450 mg PO q.i.d. Erythromycin 500mg PO b.i.d or Doxycycline 100mg PO b.i.d **Oral anaerobes**
Acute paronychia Felon	Gram-positive cocci *Staphylococcus aureus* *Streptococcus* Anaerobes	Clindamycin 450 mg PO q.i.d.	Clindamycin 450 mg PO q.i.d. or Augmentin 875 mg PO b.i.d.
Deep space infections Dorsal Subaponeurotic Collar button abscess Thenar abscess Midpalmar abscess	Gram-positive cocci *Staphylococcus aureus* *Streptococcus* Anaerobes	Clindamycin 450 mg PO q.i.d. **Inpatient Treatment** Clindamycin 900 mg IV q80	Augmentin 875 mg PO b.i.d. Bactrim DS I PO b.i.d. **Severe infections** Timentin 3.1g IV q6h or Zosyn 3.375g IV q6h or Vancomycin 1 gm IV q12h + Cefepime 1 gm IV q12h
Diabetic wounds	Polymicrobial contamination Gram-positive cocci Gram negative rods *Pseudomonas aeruginosa*	Clindamycin 450 mg PO q.i.d. + Fluoroquinolone or Ciprofloxacin 500 mg b.i.d. or Maxistone 400 mg qd **Severe infections** Extended spectrum Penicillin Timentin 3.1g IV q6h	**Severe infections** Vancomycin 1 gm IV q12h + Cefepime 1 gm IV q12h

Table 15–1 *(Continued)*

Infection Type	Organism	Antimicrobial Therapy	Alternative Therapy
Diabatic Wounds (Continued)	Zosyn 3.375 gm q6h IV	With fluoroquinolone	
Cat bites Dog bites	*Pasturella multocida*	Augmentin 875 mg PO b.i.d. Inpatient Treatment Unasyn 1.5 gm IV q6h	Penicillin allergy Clindamycin 480 mg PO q.i.d+ Ciprofloxacin 500mg PO b.i.d or Bactrim DS PO b.i.d
Human bites	*Eikenella corrodens* *Oral anaerobes* *Peptococcus* *Peptostreptococcus*	Augmentin 875mg PO b.i.d. Inpatient Treatment Unasyn 1.5 gm IV q6h	Penicillin allergy Clindamycin 480 mg PO q.i.d+ Ciprofloxacin 500mg PO b.i.d or Bactrim DS PO b.i.d
Onychomycosis	*Trichophyton rubrum* *Candida albicans*	Terbinafine 250 mg PO qd × 6 weeks	Itraconazole 200 mg PO q.d. or Fluconazole 100 mg PO q.d.
Sea water contamination	Mycobacterium marinum	Clarithromycin 250 mg PO b.i.d.	Minocycline 100 mg PO b.i.d. or Doxycycline 100 mg PO b.i.d. or Bactrim DS PO b.i.d. or RIfamopin 600 m PO q.d. + Ethambutol 120V mg PO q.d.
Necrotizing infections Flexor tenosynovitis	Polymicrobial contamination Gram positive cocci Gram negative rods Anaerobes	Vancomycin 1 gm IV q12h + Cefepime 1 gm IV q12h Clindamycin 900 mg IV q8h	Zosyn 3.375 mg IV q6h+ Moxifloxacin 400 mg IV/PO q.d.

Abbreviations: MRSA, methicillin-resistant Staphylococcus aureus.

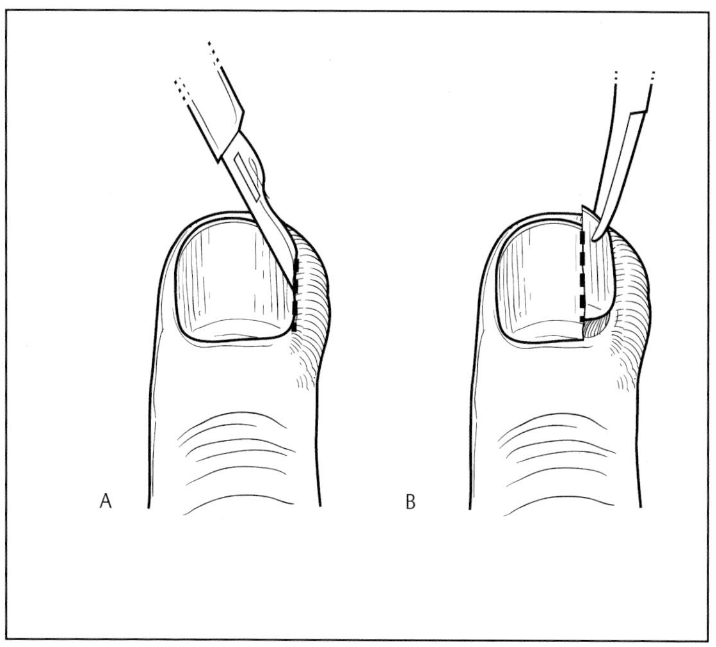

Figure 15–1 **(A)** Incision and drainage of paronychial infection. **(B)** Partial nail excision.

- Elevation
- Short-term follow-up

A paronychia that has developed purulence requires drainage:

- Perform a digital block (see Chapter 13, Fig. 13–1)
- Use the no-nail excision technique (**Fig. 15–1A**)
  - Elevate the nail fold using small elevator from the perionychial/eponychial junction to the proximal nail edge.
  - Excise the distal third of the nail to evacuate purulent material and if needed for additional exposure
- Incision technique (**Fig. 15–1B**)
  - Begin with a longitudinal incision along the lateral nail fold with a 15-blade beveled away from the nail
  - Repeat bilaterally if both sides are involved
  - Drain purulent material at the base of the nail by elevating the eponychial fold
  - Excise a longitudinal strip of the nail adjacent to the fold with an edge of the eponychium for drainage

- ◦ Extensive eponychial and subungual infections require removal of the nail plate and stenting of the fold with Iodoform garze.

Postoperative Care

- Warm soaks three times a day with a 1:1 solution of 3% hydrogen peroxide and normal saline
- Oral antibiotics for one week
- Elevation
- Short-term followup
- Avoid nail biting and trimming nails too closely

Chronic Paronychia

Chronic paronychia is defined as an infection that involves the eponychial, paronychial fold, or the nail matrix lasting longer than 6 weeks. Fungi are most commonly associated with these infections. *Candida albicans* is the primary infectious organism. However, atypical mycobacteria are implicated in hand infections of persons chronically exposed to water. Generally, these infections are found in swimmers, dishwashers, and housekeepers who have prolonged exposure to moist environments and repeated exposure to chemical irritants.

Treatment

- Topical miconazole b.i.d. or Terbinafin
- Oral ketoconazole 200 mg PO q.d. or fluconazole 100 mg PO q.d. for 4 weeks
- Consider biopsy to rule out squamous cell carcinoma for recalcitrant disease
- Marsupialization
  - Perform a digital block
  - Apply finger tourniquet
  - Using a 15-blade scalpel incise along the proximal and distal edge of the eponychium in a crescent fashion
  - Excise the eponychial skin and infected tissue leaving the germinal matrix intact
  - Irrigate the exteriorized germinal matrix, then pack the region with iodoform gauze
  - Remove the nail plate if grossly deformed
- Change the dressing every day until complete epithelialization has occurred

Felon

The volar pad of the distal phalanx is divided into 15 to 20 fibrous fascial compartments by vertical fibrous septa extending from the dermis to the distal phalanx. Infections in this area are compartmentalized, causing the formation of small abscesses. *S. aureus*, *Streptococci*, and anaerobes cause most felons. Evaluation should rule out the presence a foreign body, which occasionally can be detected radiographically. Persistent disease will result in extension to the distal phalanx and possibly the tendon sheath of the flexor digitorum superficialis (FDS), causing osteomyelitis or flexor tenosynovitis, respectively.

Treatment

The volar pad septae must be completely obtiterated, while minimizing damage to the neurovascular bundle:

- Perform a digital block
- Apply a finger tourniquet
- Mark the nondominant side of the finger for the incision. This is usually the ulnar side of the index, long finger, or ring finger. For the thumb and little finger, release via an incision on the radial side of the digit.
- Incisions
  - High lateral incision (**Fig. 15–2**)
  - Fish mouth incision
  - Palmar longitudinal incision
- Obtain culture
- Spread through septa-disrupting compartment

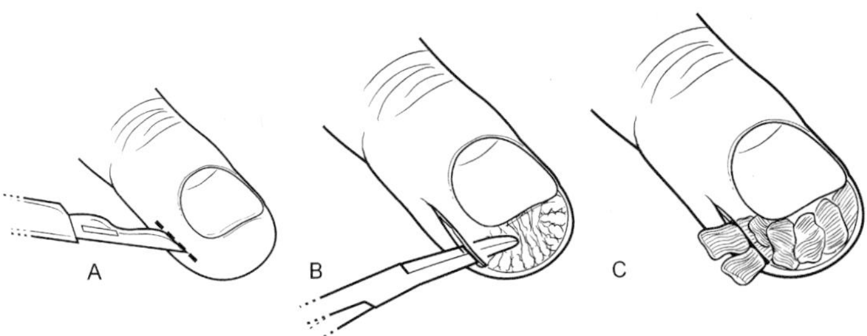

Figures 15–2 **(A)** High lateral incision avoiding neurovascular bundle **(B)** Disruption of the ventral fibrous septa **(C)** Packing of the space with Iodoform gauze after thorough irrigation.

(Continued)

D

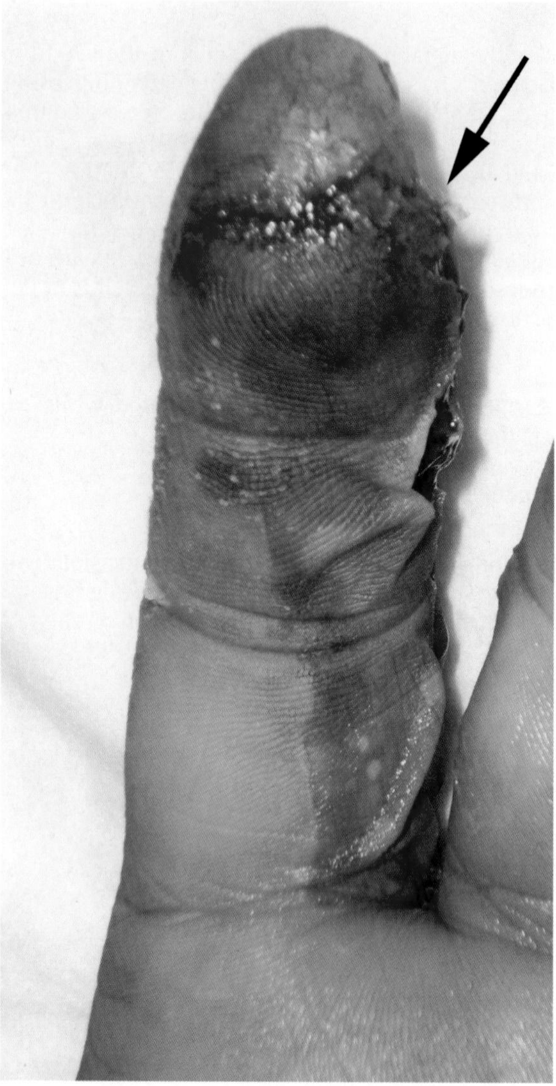

Figures 15–2 *(Continued)* **(D)** Complicated felon demonstrating epidermolysis extending to the ulnar position of the index finger.

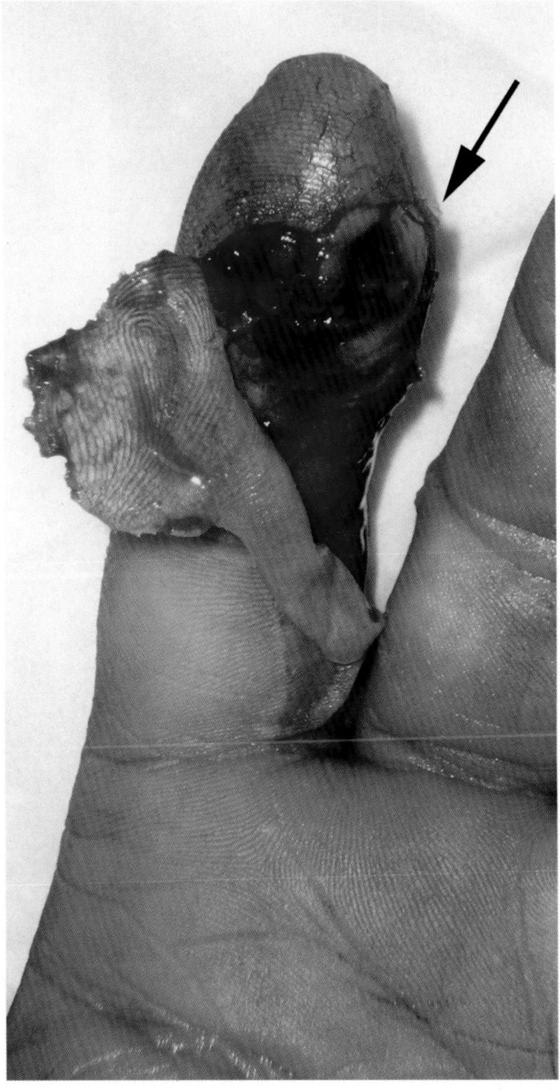

Figures 15–2 *(Continued)* **(E)** Débrietment of the detatched epidermis and ulna based incisions and drainage of felon.

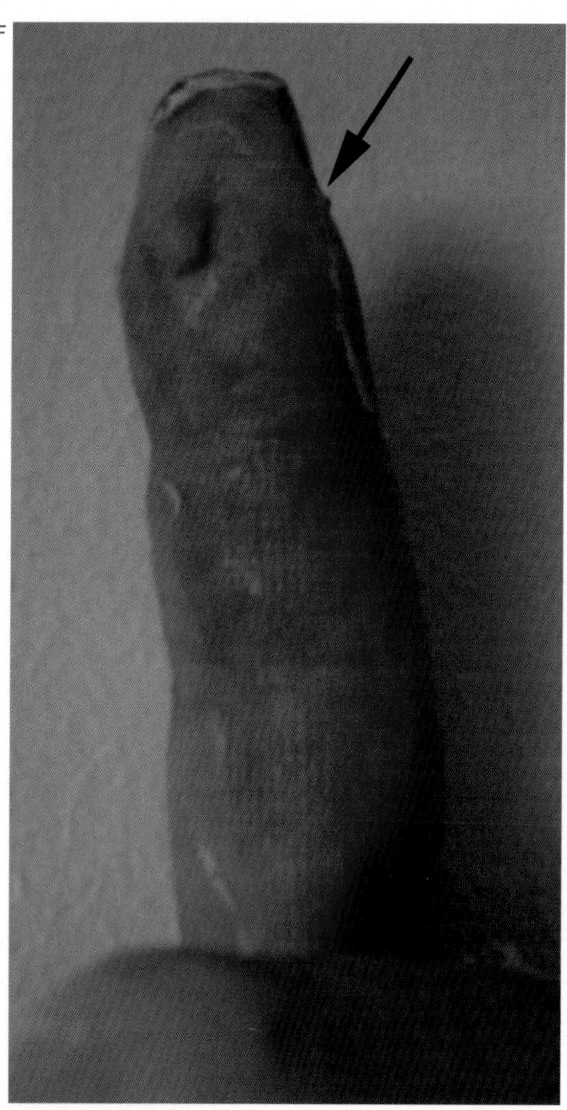

Figures 15–2 *(Continued)* **(F)** One-month postoperative follow-up. The arrow indicates site of felon.

- Irrigate thoroughly
- Pack with iodoform gauze

Postoperative Care

- Warm soaks three times a day with a 1:1 solution of 3% hydrogen peroxide and normal saline
- Oral antibiotics for one week
- Elevation
- Short-term follow-up

Herpetic Whitlow

Herpes simplex is the causative organism associated with vesicular eruption of the distal digits. The viral contamination is usually secondary to exposure to oral secretions. Health care workers, particularly dentists and anesthesiologists, are at increased risk. Physical examination reveals clear vesicles that progress to ulceration within 14 days. The volar pad is edematous, but soft and painful to palpation. Diagnosis can be confirmed by viral cultures and a Tzanck smear that demonstrates multinucleated giant cells. The ability of the virus to live in the dorsal root ganglion promotes the recurrence of this disease.

Treatment

- *Do not incise and drain*
- A self-limited disease that resolves in 10 to 14 days
- Cleanse wound twice a day to prevent a bacterial superinfection
- Cover wound with loose dressing
- Oral antiviral drugs decrease the clinical course and recurrence
  - Acyclovir 200 mg PO q4h × 10 days (recurrence × 5 days), suppression 400 mg PO b.i.d.
  - Valacyclovir 1 g PO b.i.d. × 10 days (recurrence 500 g PO b.i.d.), suppression 500 g PO q.d.

Flexor Tenosynovitis

Synovitis of the flexor tendon sheath occurs from inflammatory and infectious etiologies. In the acute setting, suppurative stenosing infection of the flexor tendon sheath requires rapid evaluation and treatment to prevent extension to the forearm. Infections of the flexor tendon sheath result from either direct extension from a subcutaneous abscess (e.g., felon, midpalmar space abscess) or direct inoculation from penetrating trauma. A patient who presents with flexor tenosynovitis will exhibit the four Kanavel signs:

Pain **On passive extension**

Tenderness Along tendon sheath

Edema Fusiform swelling of the entire digit

Flexion Fixed flexion posture at rest

The tendon sheath is a closed space from the DIP to the A1 pulley. The thumb and small finger tendon sheaths communicate with the radial and ulna bursae, respectively, and continue into the wrist. The radial and ulnar bursae communicate via the Paronas space. The intricate architecture and proximity of the tendon sheaths and bursae allow extension of the infection to the hand proximally. Additional potential complications include carpal tunnel syndrome, tendon necrosis, and tendon adhesions.

Treatment

Patients with flexor tenosynovitis require hospital admission, broad-spectrum antibiotics, and urgent operative exploration.

- Bring the patient to the operating room
- Place tourniquet and exsanguinate arm by elevating arm for 2 minutes and occluding the brachial artery. Raise tourniquet to 100 mm Hg greater than the SBP. Do not exsanguinate using mechanical exsanguination techniques
- Limited incision and catheter drainage (**Fig. 15–3D**)
  - Incise the mid-axial border of the involved distal phalanx (Avoid contact and pressure surfaces)
  - Make a separate transverse incision at the level of the A1 pulley
  - Through these incisions expose the flexor tendon sheath
    - Evacuate purulence
    - Obtain culture
    - Thoroughly irrigate both wounds
  - Insert a small catheter for irrigation into the tendon sheath – (6 Fr pediatric feeding tube)
    - Irrigate

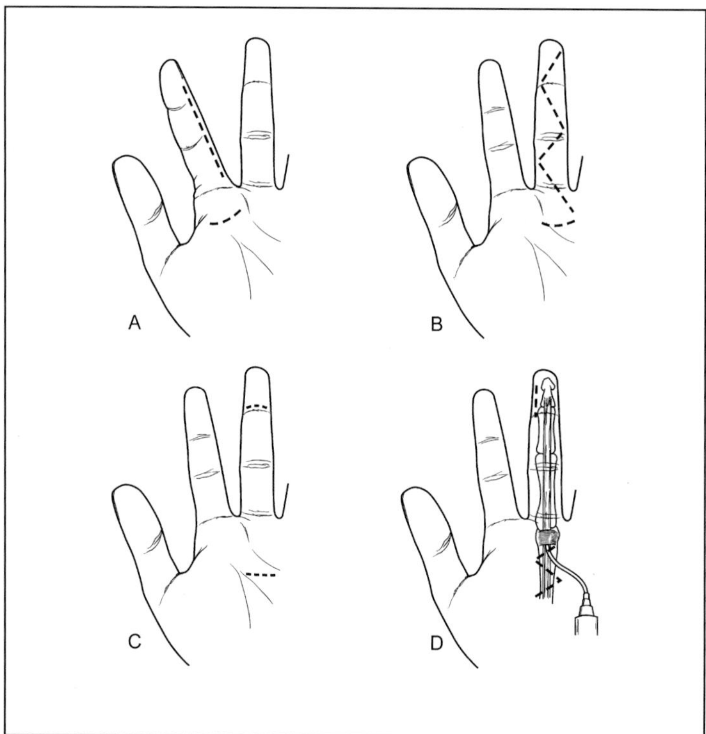

Figure 15–3 **(A–D)** Incision techniques for drainage of the flexor tendon sheath.

- Keep catheter in place for continuous irrigation
  - 500 cc normal saline + 1 g vancomycin
  - Infuse at 20 to 50 cc/hour, depending on patient tolerance
- Remove catheter in 48 hours

- Extensive exploration and débridement – required for delayed diagnosis and extensive soft tissue necrosis
  - Mark the nondominant side of the finger for the incision. This is usually the ulnar side of the index, long finger, and ring finger. For the thumb and little finger, release via an incision on the radial side of the digit.
  - Make Brunner (**Fig. 15–3B**) zigzag incisions from the distal phalanx to the palm
    - Take care not to damage the neurovascular bundles or cross the flexion creases volarly at right angles

- Evacuate purulence
  - Obtain culture
  - Remove necrotic debris
  - Thoroughly irrigate both wounds
- Close skin loosely over a small catheter for continuous catheter irrigation – 6 Fr pediatric feeding tube
  - 500 cc normal saline + 1 g vancomycin
  - Infuse at 20 to 50 cc/hour, depending on patient tolerance
  - Remove catheter in 48 hours
- Splint in safe position
- Begin ROM protocols after catheter is removed to decrease adhesions
- If there is significant soft tissue destruction, whirlpool therapy as an adjunct is useful for débridement of the devitalized soft tissues after operative drainage.

Deep Fascial Space Infections

Deep space infections begin from penetrating wounds of the hand or by extension of a superficial infection. **Figure 15–4** illustrates the anatomical relationship of the deep fascial spaces in the hand; **Fig. 15–5** shows the incisions for deep palmar abscesses.

Treatment

- Place tourniquet and exsanguinate arm by elevating arm for 2 minutes and occluding the brachial artery. Raise tourniquet to 100 mm Hg greater than the SBP
- Incision and drainage
  - The wound is left opened
  - Wound packed with iodoform or a Penrose drain is placed
  - Daily dressing changes are performed
- Small dorsal abscesses can be safely drained in the emergency room. Make incisions in between extensor tendons to avoid injury to the tendons
- Volar abscesses are explored in the operating room
- Antibiotics
- Whirlpool therapy b.i.d
  - Aids with débridement of devitalized tissue
  - Edema may be increased throughout the dumtion of therapy

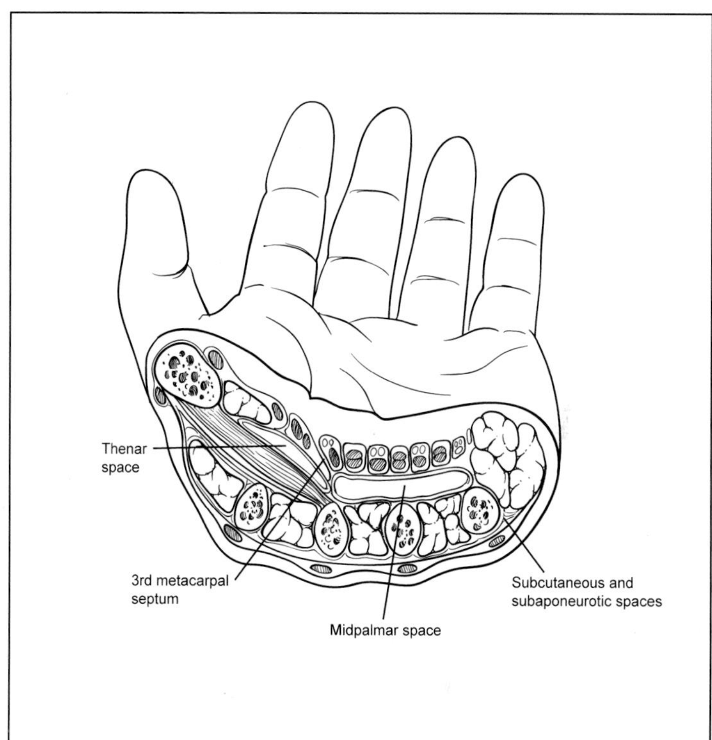

Figure 15–4 Deep fascial spaces of the hand.

Collar Button Abscess

A purulent infection of the web space is referred to as a collar button abscess. Fissures and blisters are commonly implicated as etiologies. Patients present with an hourglass configuration at the base of the digit in an abducted position. Collar button infections are drained through two longitudinal incisions on the dorsal and volar surfaces of the web space (**Fig. 15–5A**).

Dorsal Subaponeurotic and Subcutaneous Abscesses

Beneath the extensor tendons on the dorsum of the hand, an infection may reside in the subaponeurotic space, which is differentiated from an infection above the extensor tendons (subcutaneous space). Drainage is performed through longitudinal incisions. A

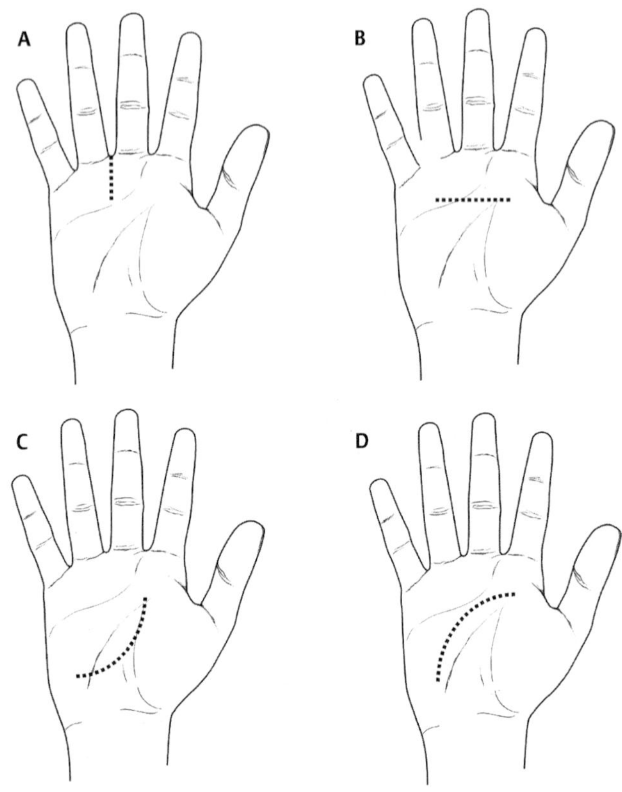

Figure 15–5 (A–D) Incision techniques for drainage of deep hand abscesses. Avoid damage to neurovascular structures.

suspected subaponeurotic infection is approached through longitudinal incisions over the index and small finger metacarpals (avoid damage to extensor tendons).

Thenar and Midpalmar Space Abscess

Thenar space infections occur in the volar soft tissues of the thumb and first dorsal interossei. The thumb is held in abduction and pain is elicited with adduction. Drainage is performed with an incision that is parallel to the thenar crease.

The midpalmar space comprises an area deep to the flexor tendons. Patients present with fluctuance, erythema, and palpable

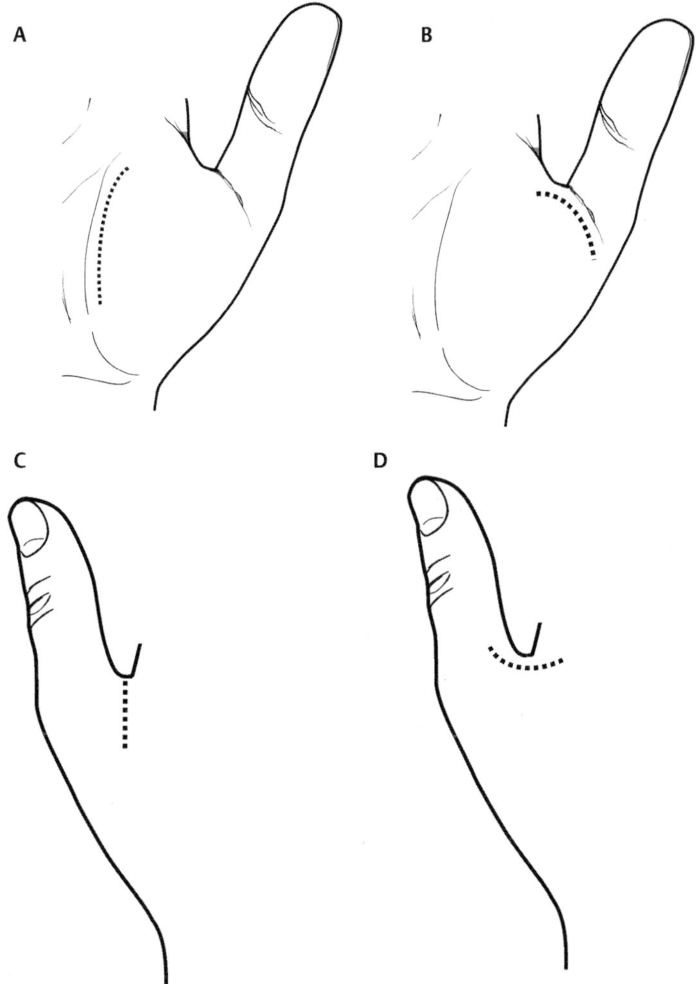

Figure 15–6 **(A–D)** Incision techniques for drainage of thenar abscesses.

tenderness in the midpalm. Transverse or oblique volar incisions are utilized to explore the flexor tendons and midpalmar space (**Fig. 15–6**). After drainage, the wounds are closed loosely over a continuous irrigation catheter.

Osteomyelitis and Septic Arthritis

Infections of the joint and bone are usually the result of open fractures, an extension of chronic soft tissue infections, or secondary to direct inoculation from a penetrating object (e.g., a tooth). Septic arthritis and osteomyelitis are less commonly the result of hematogenous contamination from a distant focus. This mechanism is particularly common in immunosuppressed and pediatric patients secondary to the intrinsic vascular architecture at the physis/epiphysis. Diagnosis is based on history and radiographic evaluation. Patients have a history of chronic infection, nonhealing wounds, or nonunions. Elevated CRP and ESR are nonspecific when acute inflammatory conditions occur simultaneously. Plain radiographs will reveal bony erosion and periosteal elevation. MRI is more specific than plain films.

Osteomyelitis is treated with débridement of the infected bone and removal of the sequestra and sinus tracts. Bone specimen is sent for pathology and culture. Antimicrobial treatment is instituted for 6 weeks.

Patients with pyogenic arthritis present with the involved joint held in a distracted position to maximize volume. Tenderness and erythema is localized over the joint. Pain is elicited with passive ROM. A subset of patients with inflammatory arthritides (e.g., gout, rheumatoid arthritis) may present with joint signs and symptoms similar to that of septic arthritis. In these cases, a careful history with serology will assist in making the diagnosis. Joint aspiration is indicated for diagnosis (**Table 15–2**) and for purposes of culture identification (**Table 15–1**). Incision and drainage of the MCP joint is performed through dorsal incisions proximal to the sagittal band. The thumb MCP joint is approached through a

Table 15–2 Diagnostic Values and Differential Diagnoses for Joint Aspirate

	Normal	Noninflammatory	Inflammatory	Septic
Volume	<3.5	>3.5	>3.5	>3.5
Clarity	Transparent	Transparent	Translucent	Opaque
WBC/ul	<200	200–300	3000–50,000	>50,000
PNMs (%)	<25%	<25%	≥50%	≥75%
Culture	Negative	Negative	Negative	Positive
Glucose (mg/dL)	=Serum	=Serum	>25, <Serum	<25, <Serum

(Continued)

Table 15–2 *(Continued)*

Noninflammatory	Inflammatory	Septic
DJD Trauma Osteochondritis dissecans Neuropathic arthropathy Subsiding or early inflammation Hypertrophic osteoarthropathy Pigmented villonodular synovitis	Rheumatoid arthritis Gout and pseudogout Reiters syndrome Ankylosing spondylitis Psoriatic arthritis UC or enteritis Scleroderma Tuberculosis Mycotic infections	Pyogenic infections

Hemorrhagic
Hemophilia Trauma Neuropathic arthropathy Pigmented villonodular synovitis Synovioma Hemangioma and other tumors

Abbreviations: PNMs, polynuclear monocytes; DJD, degenerative joint disease; UC, ulcerative coliting.

mid-axial ulnar incision. The IP joints are also approached through a mid-axial incision and irrigated with a butterfly needle.

♦ Hand Injection Injuries

These injuries occur most commonly secondary to industrial guns loaded with paints, grease, or fuels. Pressure of about 100 lb/sq in (7 kg/cm^2) is required to penetrate the epidermis, but industrial guns can inject with a power of 10 to 100 times greater than this pressure. The nondominant index finger is the most affected site.

Although the site of injection and penetration of fluids under pressure may seem small initially, most such injuries require wide surgical incision of the hand, meticulous lavage, and débridement.

Symptoms are initially subtle. At times only a small pinpoint punture in the skin. After several hours, however, patients complain of increasing edema, pain, dysesthesia, and discoloration. If left untreated, this will progress to necrosis, gangrene, lymphangitis, and bacterial infections.

Examination

- Determine the precise location of injury, the time of injury, type of fluid injected, and tetanus status vaccination.
- Examine the entire upper extremity because the superficial appearance of the injury often belies the extent of tissue damage.
- Neurovascular evaluation and documentation are essential.
- Check X-rays to rule out fractures and visualize radiographically opaque material.

Treatment

- Tetanus vaccine
- Broad-spectrum antibiotic coverage (vancomycin 1 gm IV q12h + cefepime 1 gm IV q12h or Zosyn 3.375 mg IV q60)
- Elevate limb
- Immediate surgical exploration
- Evaluate the need for fasciotomy if injury presents late

Operative Treatment

Use an upper extremity tourniquet without using mechanical exsanguination. Instead, raise the arm for 3 minutes while compressing the brachial artery prior to inflation of the tourniquet. Use an axillary block for anesthesia.

Perform Brunner (**Fig. 15–3B**) or mid-lateral (**Fig. 15–3A**) incisions in the fingers. Brunner incisions are performed by first cutting along a diagonal line from the lateral nail-bed site to the flexion crease on the opposite site. The incision is then zigzagged back diagonally to the next flexion crease on the opposite site. It can be carried proximally across the palm. A mid-lateral incision is first marked by first flexing the finger. Next, a line is drawn which interconnects the most dorsal aspect of the flexion creases to each other and to a point lateral to the nail plate. The nondominant side of the finger is usually the ulnar side of the index, long finger, and ring finger. For the thumb and little finger, release via an incision on the radial side of the digit.

Culture any purulent material that may be present. The most common infecting agent in these wounds is *Staphylococcus epidermidis* and polymicrobial infections are common. It is important to débride all nonviable tissues while preserving neurovascular structures that are not affected. Depending on the spread of the material, a carpal tunnel release may be required. In addition, open all involved tendon sheaths and the radial and ulnar bursae. Irrigate all involved structures thoroughly. Do not attempt to neutralize any chemicals because the neutralizing chemicals often cause damage. Pack the wound with wet (saline-soaked) gauze and be prepared for further débridement in the operating room if necessary 24–48 hours later. Splint the involved extremity in a safe position (see Chapter 13). If the injected material was radio-opaque, then a postoperative x-ray may help to determine if all material was removed.

Postoperative Care

Ensure the wound is clean and clear of devitalized tissue through as much débridement as necessary. Whirlpool therapy may be used postoperatively to provide additional debridement. Elevate the involved extremity when the patient is in a splint. Attempt to start activity in the extremity as soon as possible to decrease the amount of contractures. In subsequent surgeries, attempt to close parts of the wound that are clean and granulating. Use a skin graft or synthetic/acellular dermal matrix and a skin graft to close wounds. Alternatively, severely contaminated wounds can be closed by secondary intention. Begin the patient on hand/occupational therapy as soon as possible because therapy is a major determinant of the patient's ultimate level of function.

16

Hand and Forearm Tendon Injuries

Injuries of the distal upper extremity range from simple lacerations to complex open blast injuries involving destruction of vital soft tissue nerve and vascular structures. Effective evaluation and treatment requires detailed attention to the mechanism, time, and level of injury. The initial evaluation of an injured hand or forearm consists of a complete assessment for bony, vascular, and soft tissue injuries. Complex injuries mandate prioritizing reconstruction. First, the osseous structures are stabilized with internal or external fixation methods. Following rigid stabilization of the extremity, soft tissue repair is undertaken to protect and provide minimal tension over delicate vascular and nerve reconstructions. When loss of soft tissue is extensive, priority is placed on bony stabilization and revascularization. Soft tissue coverage is then employed and the soft tissue is allowed to stabilize and heal for 3 weeks. Tendon and nerve reconstruction is delayed until soft tissue coverage has stabilized.

Tendon injuries of the forearm and hand range from simple an incomplete laceration of a single tendon to maceration and structural loss of multiple musculotendenous units. The mechanism of injury dictates the method of repair. Simple tendon lacerations are repaired directly with any familiar tendon repair technique (**Fig. 16–1**). The repair of tendon lacerations that are the result of blast and avulsion injuries is usually delayed because the extent of tendon damage is not immediately known. A delay of 3 to 4 weeks allows the determination of viable tendon, at which point, tendon reconstruction with tendon grafts is performed. Over the course of the delay, the tendon path and muscle length can be preserved utilizing

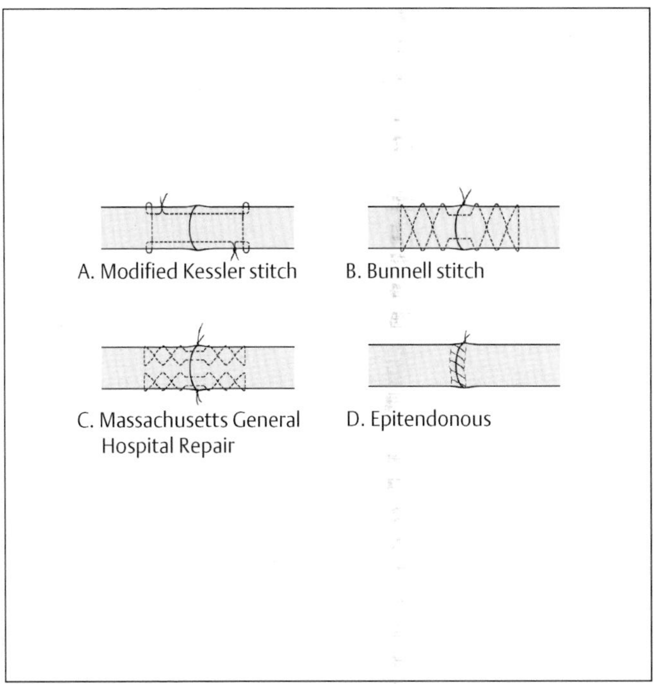

Figure 16–1 Tendon injury repairs. **(A)** Modified Kessler stitch. **(B)** Bunnell stitch. **(C)** Massachusetts General Hospital repair. **(D)** Epitendonous suture.

Silastic (Dow Corning, Midland, MI and Barry, UK) tendon rods sutured to the injured tendon ends.

♦ Extensor Tendon Injuries

Patients with extensor tendon injuries present with obvious lacerations over the involved tendon, or palpable pain in the region of a closed injury. The resting hand position will display the involved digit in flexion secondary to the loss of the counterbalancing extensor. The patient will also be unable to extend the involved digit actively while the palm of the hand is face down on a flat surface (tabletop test).

Extensor tendon injuries are commonly the result of open lacerations, but also occur secondary to a variety of closed etiologies.

Closed traumatic rupture of the extensor tendon includes but ins't limited to: rupture of the extensor tendon at distal insertion of the distal phalanx (mallet finger) or central slip from the dorsum of the middle phalanx (boutonnière deformity), and rupture of the extensor pollicis longus associated with radius fractures. Patients with rheumatoid arthritis develop attrition ruptures at multiple levels that can also present in a similar fashion.

Anatomy

The extensor compartments of the hand are separated into six dorsal compartments:

- Abductor pollicis longus and extensor pollicis brevis
- Extensor carpi radialis longus and brevis
- Extensor pollicis longus
- Extensor indicis and extensor digitorum communis
- Extensor digiti minimi (quinti)
- Extensor carpi ulnaris

Longitudinally the extensor tendon is divided into nine zones from its course from the muscle to insertion into the distal phalanx (**Fig. 16–2**):

Zone I Distal interphalangeal joint
Zone II Middle phalanx
Zone III Proximal interphalangeal joint
Zone IV Proximal phalanx
Zone V Metacarpophalangeal joint
Zone VI Metacarpal
Zone VII Carpus
Zone VIII Distal forearm
Zone IX Musculotendinous junction proximal forearm muscle

The thumb has only five zones (**Fig. 16–2**):

Zone I Interphalangeal joint
Zone II Proximal phalanx
Zone III Metacarpophalangeal joint

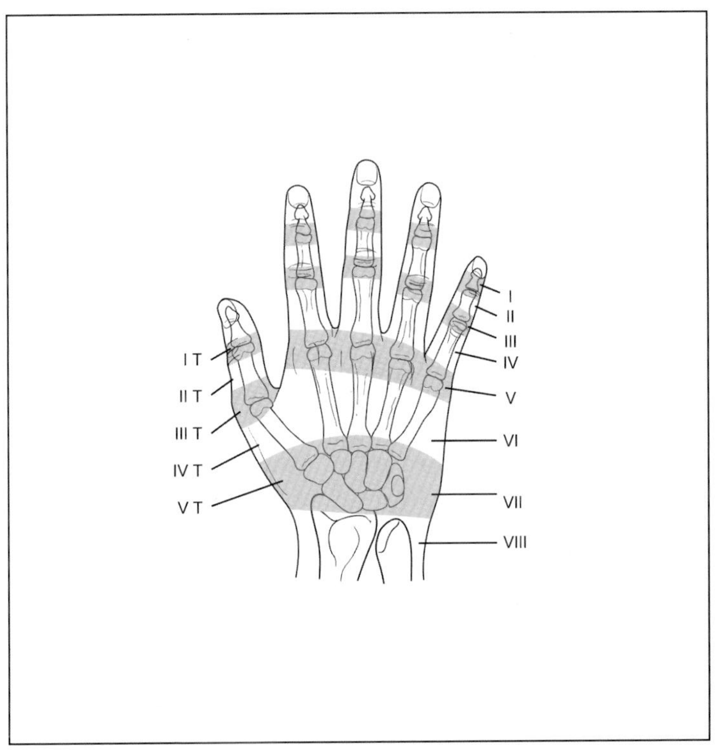

Figure 16–2 Extensor tendon zones.

Zone IV Metacarpal joint

Zone V Carpus

The extensor tendon zones are a useful tool for describing the level of injury; they also correlate to functional prognosis. For ease of reference, the odd-numbered zones are located over the joints and the even-numbered zones are located over the bone.

In the proximal forearm, the extensor digitorum communis tendons arise from a common muscle belly and disallow independent extension of the middle and ring fingers. The exceptions are the index and small fingers, which have their respective independent extensors (extensor indicis proprius, extensor digit quinti. In zone V, the juncture tendinea connect the long, ring, and small finger tendons allowing ~30 degrees of flexion of the MCP joint even if the specific extensor digit to that tendon is cut. This anatomical configuration may confuse physical examination findings when obvious lacerations suggest proximal injury.

Timing of Repair

The timing of a repair depends primarily on the extent of the injury. Simple extensor tendon lacerations may be repaired easily in the emergency room with adequate local anesthesia. However, complex injuries of multiple tendons at many levels or with gross contamination require repair in the operating room, which allows the patient the benefit of sustained anesthesia in a tourniquet-controlled environment. Tendon injuries that are not associated with ischemic-related injury to the hand or digit are repaired within one week. If it is not feasible to repair the tendon at the initial evaluation, the wound is irrigated and temporarily closed and the patient is placed in a volar splint with wrist, MP, and IP joints in slight extension.

Treatment

Due to the complex architecture of the extensor tendon, the treatment regimen and aftercare is dependant on area of injury. Generally, complete open lacerations are repaired acutely, while closed and partial (<50%) injuries can be treated with appropriate splinting to allow healing.

Zone 1

Mallet deformities are classified into four types:

Type I Closed laceration with or without fracture of the distal phalanx (less than one third of the articular surface)
Type II Open injury without fracture of the distal phalanx
Type III Open injury with loss of skin and subcutaneous cover
Type IV Fracture of the distal phalanx involving one third or more of the articular surface

Closed mallet deformities (type I) are treated by splinting the DIP joint in extension for 6 weeks. The splint is isolated to the DIP joint and spares the PIP joint. Open injuries are repaired by dermotenodesis. The skin and tendon are repaired in a composite fashion with mattress or continuous 4–0 monofilament nonabsorbable sutures.

The combination of K-wire fixation of the DIP joint in extension for 6 weeks is advocated in type III/IV injuries. K-wire fixation of the DIP joint should also be considered in all pediatric zone I extensor tendon injuries because of the high incidence of noncompliance with splinting.

Zone II

Dermotenodesis is also recommended in this zone with mattress or continuous 4–0 monofilament nonabsorbable sutures for open injuries.

Zone III

Injuries at the PIP joint level involve the central slip and lateral bands. Disruption of the central slip causes volar displacement of the lateral bands. This results in a configuration in which the PIP joint is fixed in flexion and the DIP joint is fixed in extension: the boutonnière deformity. Closed injuries at this level may not be clinically apparent in the initial period after injury and usually develop 2 to 3 weeks after central slip rupture secondary to progressive migration of the lateral bands.

Closed acute boutonnière deformity is treated with either splinting of the PIP joint in full extension or K-wire fixation of the PIP joint in extension. Splintage places the PIPJ in maximum extension with the MP and DIP joints free for six weeks. Active and passive ROM is encouraged in the DIP joint while the PIP joint is held static in extension. Open injuries of the central slip or lateral bands are repaired directly. The lateral bands are repaired with 5–0 or 6–0 monofilament nonabsorbable mattress sutures. Complete laceration of the central slip is repaired with 4–0 monofilament nonabsorbable modified Kessler or Bunnell sutures. The patient is then splinted with the wrist in 15 to 30 degrees extension and the MP and PIP joints in full extension.

Obliquely placed K-wires across the PIPJ is a reliable way to hold the joint in firm extension for closed injuries or in complexes cases of soft tissue loss. K-wires are utilized for three weeks, then removed and the patient is placed in a PIPJ extension splint wih the MP and DIP joints free, similar to that described above for an additional three weeks.

Zones IV and V

The extensor tendon over the MP joint and the proximal phalanx is composed of the central slip and the sagittal bands. At this level, injuries of the extensor tendon are not only associated with open injures, but also closed injuries secondary to forceful flexion or extension. This is most common in the middle finger and is usually secondary to a tear of the radial sagittal band. Rupture of the radial or ulnar sagittal bands causes contralateral subluxation of the central slip. Physical examination reveals incomplete finger extension with unilateral displacement of the tendon.

The central slip is repaired primarily with 4–0 monofilament nonabsorbable modified Kessler or Bunnell sutures. The sagittal bands are repaired with 5–0 monofilament nonabsorbable horizontal mattress sutures. In cases in which there is loss of substance of the sagittal band mechanism, the tendon should be centered on the MP joint by either suturing the transverse fibers to the joint capsule or tethering the tendon with the juncturae tendinum or a retrograde slip of the tendon. Splinting in these zones after repair is with the wrist in 45 degrees extension, the MP joint in 15 degrees flexion, and the PIP joints in full extension.

Open injuries in zone V are also associated with human bites, the so-called fight bite wound. In this case, the contaminated wound should be explored and the joint inspected if the capsule is violated. The wound is then cultured, thoroughly irrigated, and left open. The associated tendon laceration is repaired secondarily in 5 to 7 days, depending on the status of the surrounding soft tissue. The patient is treated with Augmentin (GlaxoSmithKline, Mississauga, Ontario, Canada) 875 mg twice a day (clindamycin for penicillin-allergic patients) for 10 days. Patients that present with an obvious infection after a human bite injury are admitted and placed on Unasyn (Pfizer Pharmaceuticals, New York, NY).

Zones VI and VII

Tendon injuries in these zones are usually secondary of open lacerating injuries. Fortunately, these injuries have the best prognosis due to the well-defined tendon substance and nourishing paratenon. Tendons are repaired in these regions with four-stranded core sutures with the knots buried and an epitendinous suture. A modified Kessler suture with a 3–0 looped Supramid (S. Jackson, Inc., Alexandria, VA) suture will facilitate four core sutures with one knot. The epitendinous repair is performed with a 6–0 continuous nylon suture. In zone VII, the extensor retinaculum is partially excised longitudinally over the repair to provide adequate excursion and to prevent formation of adhesions. Repairs in this zone are splinted with the wrist 45 degrees in extension, the MP joint in 15 degrees flexion, and the PIP joints in full extension.

Zones VII and VIII

Proximal and distal forearm injuries to extensor compartments of the forearm occur from the extensor origin at the lateral epicondyle to the wrist. In the proximal forearm, lacerations involve the muscle belly of the involved digit extensor. These injuries commonly include laceration of the radial sensory nerve and significant hematoma. Penetrating wounds in this region are explored under tourniquet, irrigated, and all hematoma is evacuated. Repair of the muscle belly repair with 3–0 PDS (Ethicon, Somerville, NJ) figure-eight sutures.

In the distal forearm, lacerations occur in the distal muscle belly, musculotendinous junction, or just proximal to wrist. At the junction of the tendon and muscle, the fascial margins are identified within the muscle and sutured to the distal tendon end using a 3–0 looped Supramid-modified Kessler suture. The fascial margins are repaired around the junction with a 4–0 PDS suture. Injuries more distal to this region are repaired similarly to zones VI and VII lacerations.

The extremity is splinted in an elbow immobilizing fashion after repair for 4 weeks. The elbow is placed in 90 degrees flexion, wrist in 45 degrees extension, MP joints in 15 degrees flexion, and IP joints in full extension.

♦ Flexor Tendon Injuries

Patients that present with flexor tendon damage will have disruption of the normal resting arcade. The loss of one or both flexor tendons will result in unbalanced extension of the involved digit. Usually lacerations will give clues to the level of injury. Deep lacerations of the volar surface of the finger and hand not only place the superficialis and profundus tendons at risk, but neurovascular injury should be suspected as well. A thorough examination of these patients includes radiographs, sensory evaluation, and isolated motor testing of the superficialis and profundus tendons (see Chapter 14, Fig.). Isolated injury to one flexor tendon may still allow flexion of the digits at the PIP joint. Therefore, to test the integrity of the profundus tendon the PIP joint is held in extension while flexion of the DIP joint is initiated.

Flexor Tendon Injury Zones

The area of the volar hand is divided in five zones that describe flexor tendon injuries (**Fig. 16–3**):

Zone I Distal to the insertion of the flexor digitorum superficialis (FDS)

Zone II "No man's land"; distal palmar crease to zone I

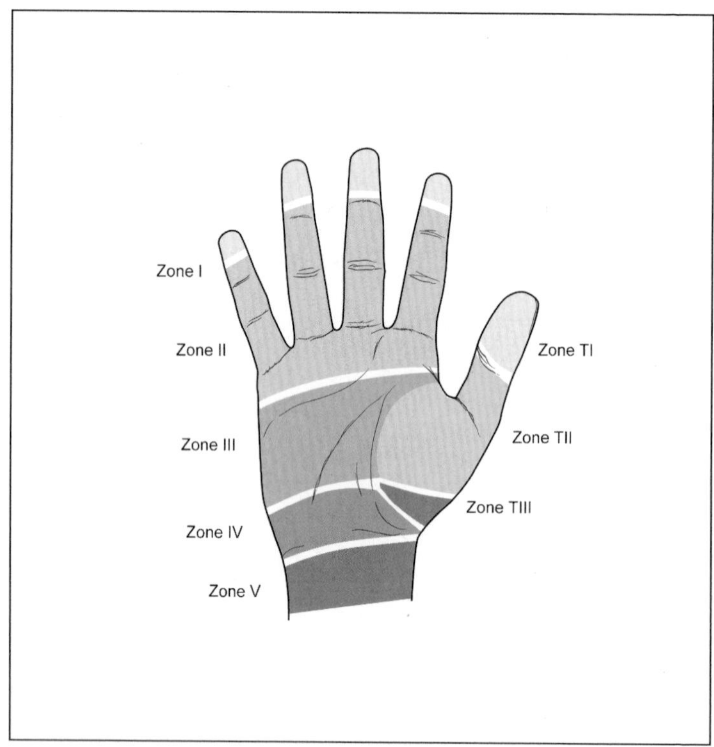

Figure 16–3 Flexor tendon zones. TI, TII and TIII are the flexor tendon zones of the thumb.

Zone III Distal edge of the transverse carpal ligament to the distal palmar crease

Zone IV The carpal tunnel

Zone V Distal portion of the forearm

Flexor Tendon Repair (Fig. 16–1)

- Perform repair within 48 to 72 hours
- Acutely place patient in extension block splint (see Chapter 13, Fig. 13–6)
- Delay tendon repair until bony stabilization and soft tissue decontamination
- Delay tendon repair when infection is present
- Perform tendon repair in the operating room to allow greater exposure for tendon retrieval
- Repair both the FDS and the flexor digitorum profundus (FDP) when injured
- Extension block splint after repair

Techniques for tendon retrieval:

- Flex wrist and MCP joint to advance tendon
- Mobilize proximal end with a suction catheter
- Massage proximal end into wound using an esmarch or manually
- Grab end with 18-gauge needle or skin hook
- Suture tendon end to rubber catheter to pass under pulleys or into tendon sheath

Zone I Repair

Repair of the FDP tendon distal to the insertion of the FDS takes into consideration the status of the insertion of the tendon onto the base of the distal phalanx. If an avulsion fragment is present with the FDP attached, the repair is performed with composite pin fixation of the tendon to the distal phalanx. When the FDP is detached, the distal portion is secured to the distal phalanx with a bone suture anchor (3–0 or 4–0) or pulled through the distal phalanx using a double-armed 3–0 Supramid suture and tied over a button.

In the repair of more proximal zone I injuries, the proximal tendon is retracted into the region of the middle phalanx. The distal stump that is attached to the distal phalanx is exposed by dissection of the A5 pulley. Care should be taken not to disrupt the A4 pulley. A core suture is placed in the proximal tendon end (3–0 Supramid), the needle is passed under the A4, pulled, and sutured into the distal tendon stump.

Zone II Repair

Due to the technical difficulty of repair and poorer functional outcomes, this zone is colloquially known as "no man land." Exposure for repair of zone II flexor tendon injuries requires wide exposure with proximal and distal Brunner incisions as well as dissection of the flexor tendon sheath and pulley system. The A2 and A4 pulleys should be preserved during dissection. Once the proximal tendon end is identified, a core suture (3–0 Supramid) is placed and pulled under the pulleys so that repair can be performed between a pulley sheath window. The proximal end can be held tension free by placing an 18-gauge needle in the end through the pulley and the sheath. Repair is then performed with 4–core sutures and an epitendinous 6–0 running Prolene (Ethicon, Somerville, NJ). Extreme care is taken in zone II to provide a repair that is flat without fraying to avoid tethering during tendon excursion. Partial resection of the adjacent pulley is acceptable to allow excursion of the repair.

Zones III, IV, and V

Injuries proximal to zone II have an improved prognosis with good functional recovery. However, in these zones there is a higher propensity to injure tendons of multiple digits and major nerve and vascular structures of the hand. Repair in these zones is aided with the use of extending palmar and forearm incision for exposure and tendon retrieval. Place a tourniquet on the patient's upper extremity to achieve hemostasis. The tourniquet should be raised to 100 mmhg above the systolic blood pressure. It can be left on for 2 hours, but needs to be deflated for 20 minutes prior to re-inflation for 2 more hours (5 minutes of deflation for every 30 minutes of inflation). If the patient has had a significant ischemic time >4–6 hours, then prophylactic fasiotomies may be required (chapter 19).

Always flex the interphalangeal joints, MCP joint and the wrist to deliver the distal ends of the lacerated tendons into the operative field. The lacerated ends of the wound can be extended proximally and distally to allow for exposure of the tendons, nerve and vessels. Any bone fixation should proceed any repair of soft tissues, as described in chapter 17. Identify all the flexor tendon ends. Often times, tendons are hidden in a small hematoma in the tendon sheath. Dissect out all the tendons and identify their function by pulling on the ends and noting their action. Next, tag them by performing tendon repair on the distal end of the tendon, with looped supermid sutures (Figure 16–1; we use the modified Kessler technique). Once all the ends are accounted for, match them to the proximal ends of the tendons, based on the position of the tendon ends in the proximal forearm. Having accounted for and match all the distal tendons to their counterpart in the forearm, begin repairing the tendon by completing the repair from the deepest tendon to the most superficial. Remember to perform epitendonous repair with 6.0 proline suture (Figure 16–1) after the core suture repair. If required, perform revasculrization of the hand by anastomoses of the severed ends of he ulnar or radial artery along with the cephalic vein or the veinae comitantes. Finally, repair the median or ulnar nerve injuries. These, repairs should involve lining up the fascicles and vasoneurium in the nerve and performing epineural repair using 9.0 nylon suture. The repair can be wrapped with 3-4mm neurogen tubing, if desired. All attempts should be made at primary repair, since this technique heralds the best prognosis. Mobilize the nerve to allow tension-free repair.

17

Hand Vascular Injuries and Digit Amputations

Vascular injuries of the hand and digit amputation can result in complete loss of function of the hand. These injuries require immediate attention by a specialist to ensure optimum functional results for the patient.

♦ Vascular System of the Hand

Vascular competency defines the hand's capacity to counter the stress placed on hand tissue. If a given stress outstrips the ability of the vasculature to compensate for the hand's cellular metabolic needs, vascular insufficiency results.

The hand is supplied with blood by the ulnar artery and the radial artery. New studies have demonstrated that the radial artery is dominant 57% of the time, whereas the ulnar artery is dominant 21.5% of the time (the two arteries are codominant the remaining 21.5% of the time [this topic is still controversial]). The radial artery divides into a small superficial palmar artery and large dorsal radial branch. The ulnar artery divides into superficial and deep branches. Next, the dorsal radial branch gives off the princeps pollicis and radial digital index branch and then anastomoses to the deep branch of the ulnar artery to form the deep palmar arch. The superficial branch of the radial artery anastomoses to the superficial ulnar artery to make the superficial palmar arch. The common digital arteries arise from the superficial arch. The digital branches arise from the common digital arteries. The vascular supply is regulated by metabolic demands, sympathetic tone, hormonal factors, and environmental factors.

Physical Examination

Basic tenets of the vascular examination of the hand include testing each digit for capillary refill, sensation, edema, color, gangrene, and petechiae. To test the proximal blood supply, take the blood pressure in both arms for a difference comparison. Next, perform an Allen's test (see Chapter 12). If you cannot feel a pulse, then check the wrist for radial and ulnar Doppler ultrasound signals and use Doppler ultrasonography to perform an Allen's test. Test the integrity of the palmar arches. If you are having difficulty performing a capillary refill test on the digits due to ecchymosis or avulsion of skin, you may use Doppler ultrasonography to determine the integrity of the digital vessels. For continuous monitoring of the perfusion to a finger, a pulse oximeter may be used on the involved finger.

If you are unable to perform the above exam or if the zone of injury to the vessels is in question, then an angiogram may be helpful. Finally, make sure to palpate the compartments of the forearm/hand as well as measure the compartment pressures with a Stryker needle or arterial line to rule out compartment syndrome and the need for a fasciotomy (see Chapter 19, Fig. 19–2, 19–3).

Arterial Injuries

Presentation Pallor, lack of capillary refill or pulse distally, pulsatile bleeding. Intimal damage may present with late thrombosis.

Mechanism Crush, stab, or avulsion injuries

The indications for repair of radial/ulnar artery injuries are

- Absolute indication: Hand or digital ischemia
- Relative indication: Improved cold intolerance, provide better circulation for wound healing
- Digital vessel repair: Digit ischemia

Treatment

Forearm and Hand Injuries

In cases of sharp injuries to the artery, direct repair can be performed. When there has been a crush injury to the artery or an avulsion, resection of the injured portion and the use of vein grafts for reconstruction is required. Signs of vessel damage include telescoping of the vessels, petechial hemorrhages on the vessel wall, vessel thrombosis, cobwebs in the vessels, or poor flow from proximal end of the injury. In these cases, reversed vein grafts can be used. The dorsal hand veins can serve as a good donor site. If the patient requires extensive forearm fracture reduction prior to repair of the artery, Silastic (Dow Corning, Midland, MI and Barry, UK) shunts can be used as a temporary way to reperfuse the hand until the fracture is stabile. Then arterial reconstruction is performed at that setting. A forearm fasciotomy should be performed if the patient has compartment syndrome or compartment syndrome is anticipated.

Digital Arteries

It is important to note that only one digital artery is required for adequate blood flow. In fact, digital revascularization is 90% successful. However, providing a venous outflow is critical.

Cannulation Injuries

A vessel injury can often occur from cannulation of the radial artery with an arterial line or arterial blood gas sampling. This can result in pseudoaneurysm formation, thrombosis, or arteriovenous fistula formation. The rate of thrombosis in the vessel is directly correlated to the duration of cannulation. If the patient has a loss of radial pulse, but does not have any digital ischemia, surgery is not needed. The treatment of these injuries entails surgical exploration and thrombectomy with direct arterial repair. Significant vessel gaps are repaired via reversed vein grafts harvested from the cephalic or saphenous veins. An arteriogram may be beneficial preoperatively or intraoperatively to identify the level and character of occlusion.

Hypothenar Hammer Syndrome

Hypothenar hammer syndrome, the most common cause of thrombosis in the upper extremity, results from repetitive trauma to the ulnar artery caused by the patient using his or her hand as a hammer. This syndrome usually occurs in laborers in their 50s who smoke. There is damage to the elastic lamina of the ulnar artery and either a thrombus and/or aneurysm can result. The thrombus may embolize.

The patient should refrain from the activity causing the trauma and should stop smoking. Hypothenar hammer syndrome may be treated medically with thrombolytics (urokinase, streptokinase, TPA). Alternatively, thrombectomy or resection of the involved portion of the vessel is required with either primary closure or with reconstruction using vein grafts from the forearm saphenous vein or dorsal foot). In some cases ligation of the artery allows for vasodilation and collateral flow. Keep a high index of suspicion for compartment syndrome.

♦ Digit Amputation

Replantation

Whereas revascularization of a digit refers to restoration of blood supply to an incompletely severed digit, replantation refers to reattachment and restoration of blood supply to a completely severed digit.

Indications for Replantation

- Amputation of the thumb, multiple digit amputation
- Partial hand amputation, wrist or distal forearm amputation, above the elbow amputation
- Any amputation in a child <12 years old

Relative Indication

- Single digit amputation distal to the insertion of the flexor digitorum superficialis (FDS)

Contraindications

- If the severed digit has undergone warm ischemia for >12 hours or cold ischemia for >24 hours
  - In the case of amputations proximal to the wrist, only a warm ischemia time of 6 hours and a cold ischemia of 12 hours can be tolerated.

- Successful replantation of digits with longer ischemia time has been reported.
  - If the patient is not stable medically to undergo a long operation
  - Relative contraindication: mentally unstable patients, smokers, and patients with diabetes mellitus

Crush and avulsion injuries can be expected to have a higher failure rate for replantation. If a patient presents with a severely mangled digit with multiple levels of injury, replantation will likely be unsuccessful. Another predictor or poor outcome is the presence of a redline on the skin and on the neurovascular bundles.

Preoperative Considerations

The amputated digit or part should be transported to the emergency room wrapped in a saline-soaked sponge, placed in a plastic bag, and placed on top of ice. Do not let the finger freeze or be submerged in ice because frostbite will result. Take x-rays and photographs of the hand along with the amputated digit to determine the level of injury. Prior to replantation, the amputated part should be examined under a loupe or microscopic magnification to establish the integrity of the involved vessels. Use this information to determine if replantation is feasible.

Provide good fluid resuscitation for the patient and discuss the risks and benefits of the surgery with the patient so they can understand the procedure, the need for rehabilitation, and have realistic expectations.

In the operating room, first, the bone is shortened and fixed with a K-wire, and then the repair is undertaken in the following order: extensor tendons, dorsal veins, dorsal skin, flexors, arteries, and nerves. The sequence of veins, arteries, and flexor tendons is controversial. Vessel repair and anastomoses should be performed outside of the zone of injury. The liberal use of vein grafts and venous flow-through flaps will allow microsurgical repair in a region with minimal inflammation. If multiple digits are replanted at the same time replantation should proceed part by part instead of finger by finger (i.e., same replantation step for each finger at the same time).

Postoperatively, splint the injury, place the patient is comfortable in warm room, and elevate the extremity. Leeches can be used to aid with venous congestion by providing the local anticoagulant hirudin and removal of blood. Usually the leeches are placed on the fingertip and they are engorged in 30 minutes. The therapy is performed for 5 to 7 days. Prophylactic antibiotics such as third-generation cephalosporins or gentamycin or bactrim can be used to avoid infection with *Aeromonas hydrophila*.

The best results are achieved with thumb, wrist, and distal FDS replants. Overall viability is reported at 80 to 90%.

Complications

- Cold intolerance
- Nonunion
- Malunion
- Joint contractures
- Infection

Fingertip Injuries

Tip avulsions and amputations are a subset of injuries that occur distal to the terminal arborization of the digital vessels. In this region of the distal phalanx, the digital arteries and veins are unable to be repaired microsurgically. Additionally, these injures commonly occur with concomitant nail avulsion and distal phalangeal fractures (tuft fractures). Repair of tip injuries requires attention to fracture reduction, nail repair, and soft tissue restoration.

Nail Repair

Nail anatomy is depicted in **Fig. 17–1**. Commonly after injury, patients will present with subungual hematomas that indicate disruption of the sterile matrix. Small subungual hematomas (<40% of the nail) are treated with aspiration of the subungual space and subsequent irrigation with an 18- or 20-gauge needle. When severe damage to the sterile matrix is suspected or larger subungual hematomas are present, removal of the nail plate and direct repair of the matrix is appropriate.

Complete nail plate avulsion injuries are repaired first by direct closure of sterile matrix with 6–0 plain gut suture. Next, the germinal matrix is stented with a piece of fine gauze, foil, or the native nail plate with two vertical mattress 5–0 chromic sutures. Preservation of the germinal matrix will prevent synechia and

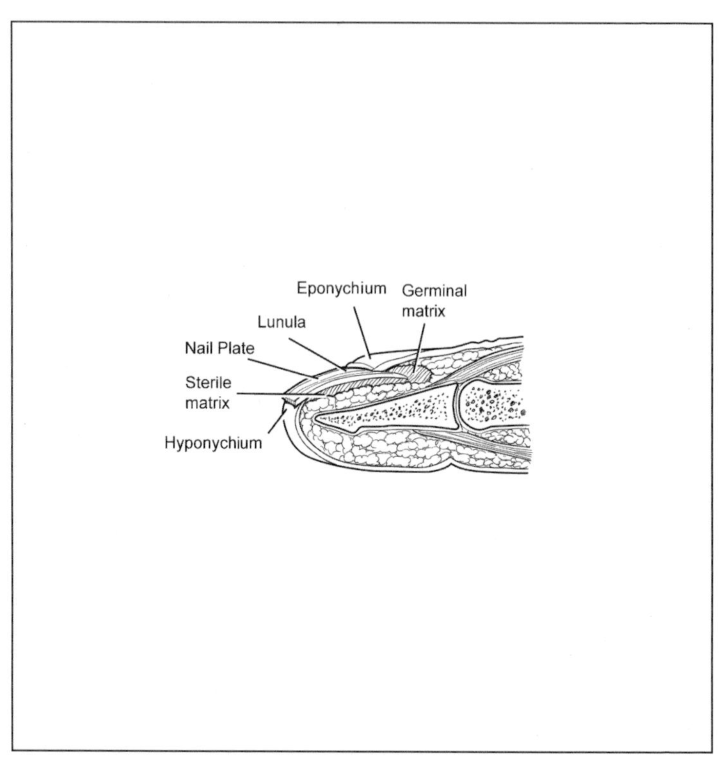

Figure 17–1 Normal fingertip anatomy.

allow growth of a new nail plate (**Fig. 17–2**). Patients should be counseled that with time the stent will be replaced by the growth of the new nail plate from beneath.

Tuft Fractures

The management of distal phalanx fractures is discussed extensively in Chapter 14. Tuft fractures occurring with tip injuries are simple and uncomplicated. Restoration of the normal soft tissue architecture by suturing and subsequent immobilization with an aluminum finger splint is adequate stabilization. The insertion of an axial K-wire or 20-gauge needle is also useful to reduce the fracture fragments.

Soft Tissue Repair

Repair of the fingertip soft tissues depends on the degree of injury (amputation vs. avulsion) and the availability of the amputated part. When avulsion of the tip is apparent, assess the avulsed fragment to determine its viability. If the avulsed fragment is cyanotic or ischemic, the fragment is amputated. If the avulsed fragment is viable, it is because the intact arterial capillary plexus between the tip and the fragment is providing perfusion. In these cases, the avulsed fragment is repaired by a suture to the tip with 4–0 nylon (5–0 chromic in children).

A primary or secondarily amputated tip can be salvaged by removing the subcutaneous tissue from the overlying glabrous skin. The skin is then sutured to the tip as a full thickness skin graft (**Fig. 17–3**). The injury is splinted and protected with an aluminum splint in place for 5 days.

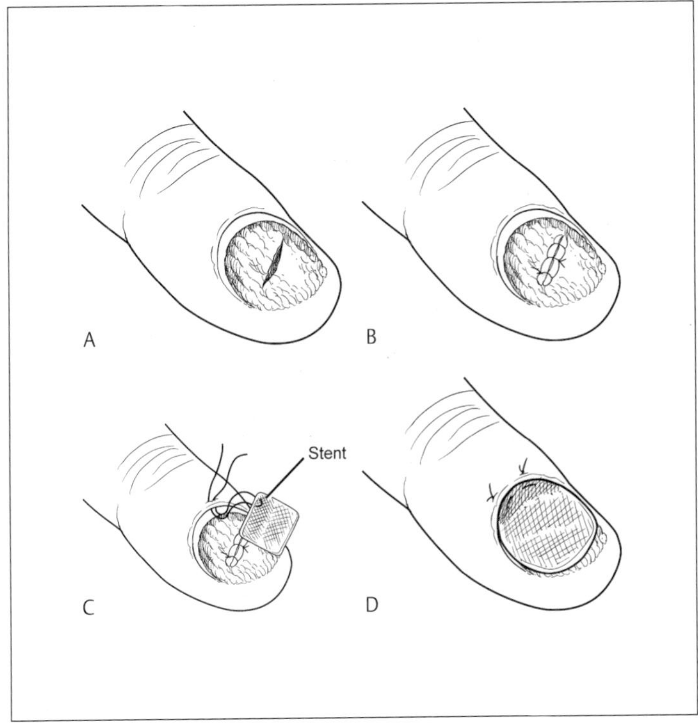

Figure 17–2 Nail bed repair. **(A,B)** Suture repair of sterile matrix laceration. **(C,D)** Germinal matrix stenting.

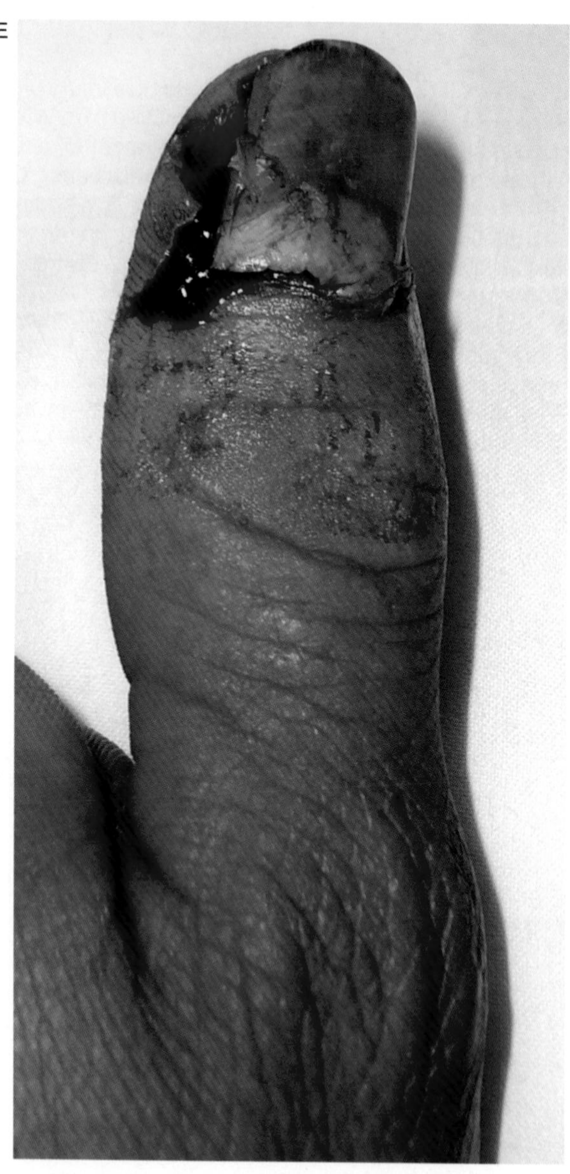

Figure 17–2 *(Continued)* **(E–H)** Repair of nail bed in a patient with distal tuft fracture.

(Continued)

F

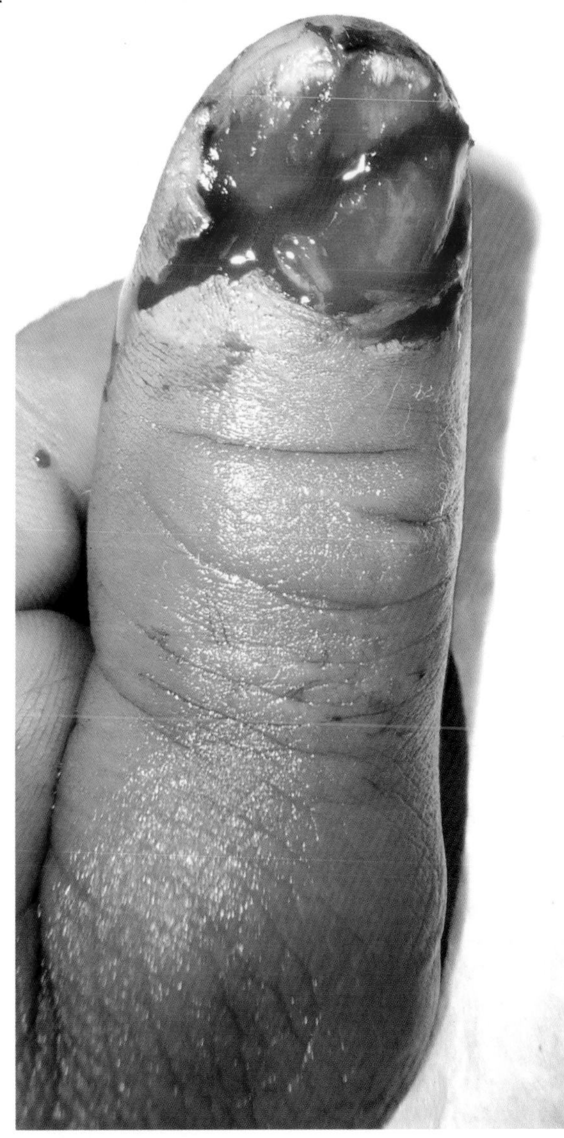

Figure 17–2 *(Continued)*

G

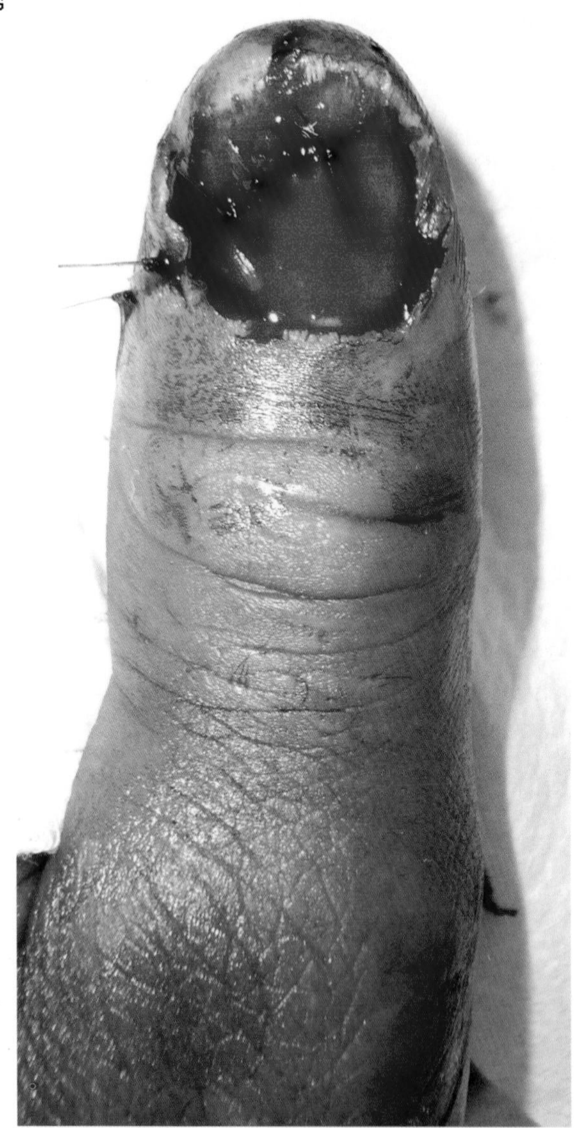

Figure 17–2 *(Continued)*

(Continued)

H

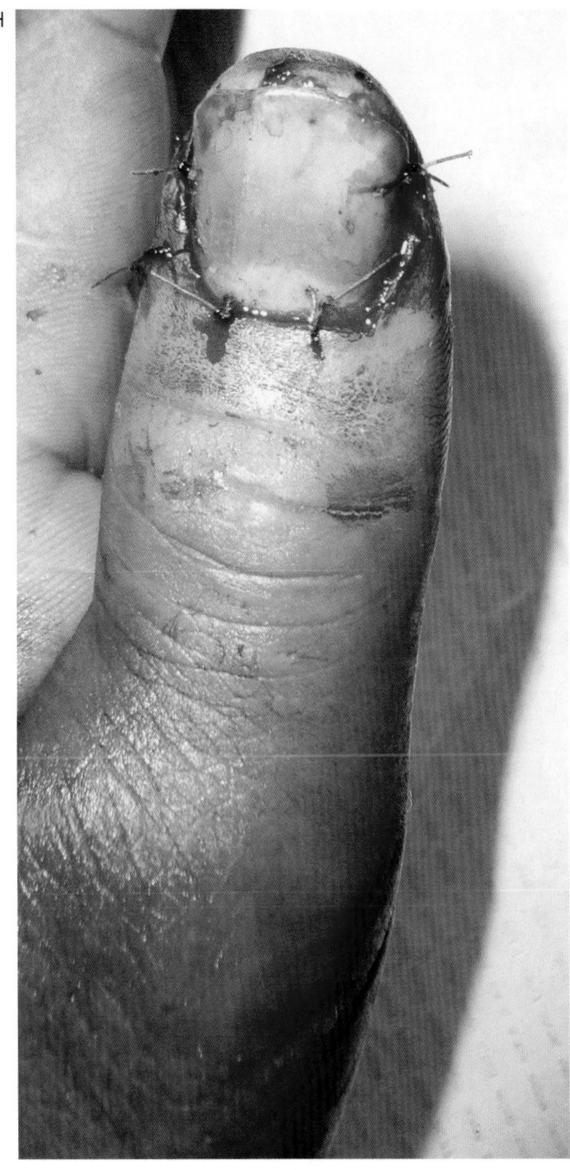

Figure 17–2 *(Continued)*

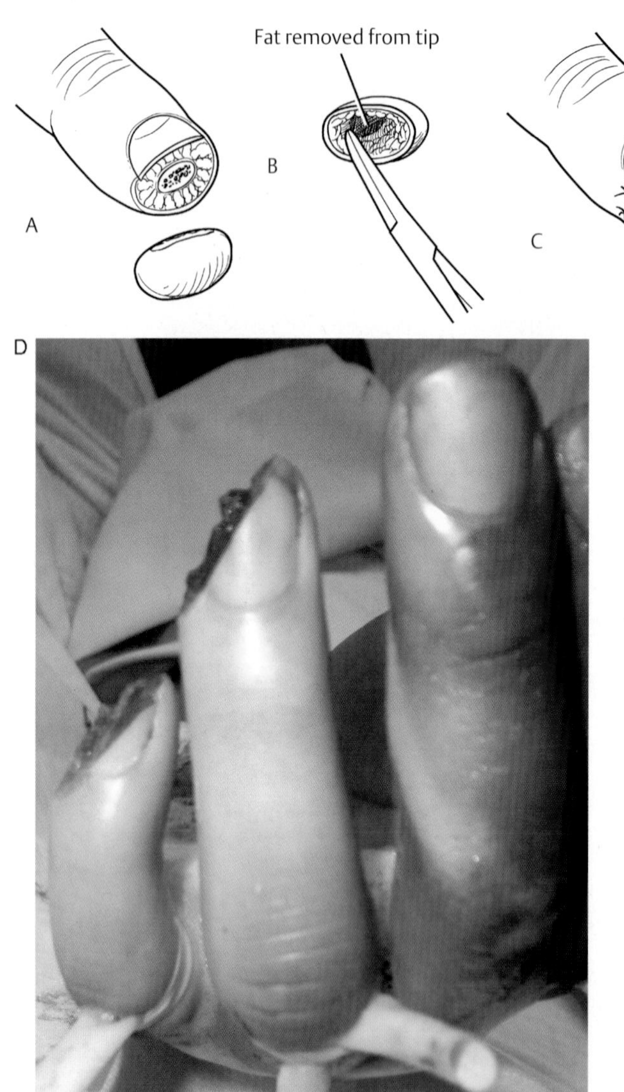

Figure 17–3 **(A–C)** Composite repair of tip amputation with amputated portion placed as a full thickness skin graft. **(D)** Presentation of distal amputation.

(Continued)

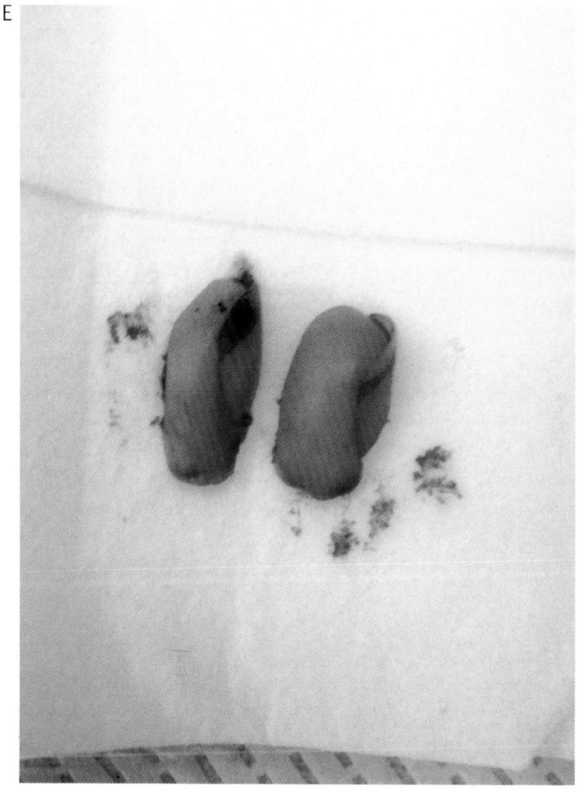

Figure 17–3 *(Continued)* **(E)** Amputated distal tuft.

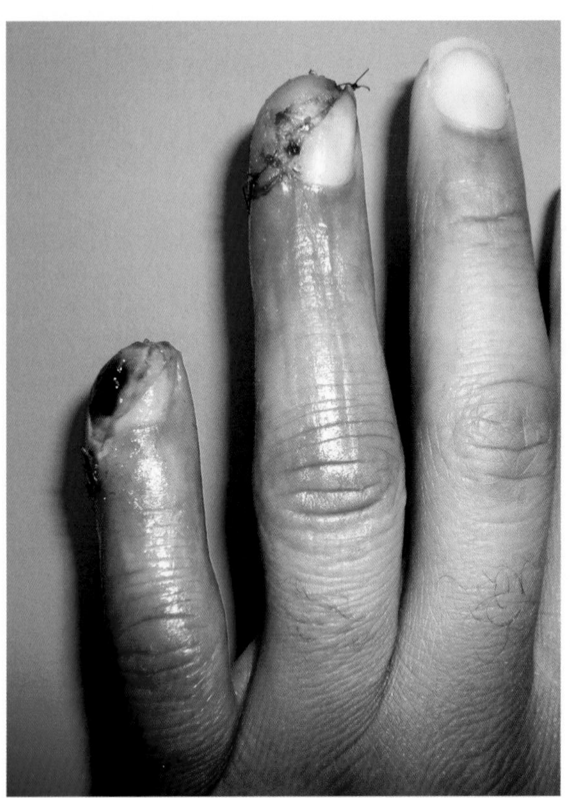

Figure 17–3 *(Continued)* **(F)** 2 weeks postrepair.

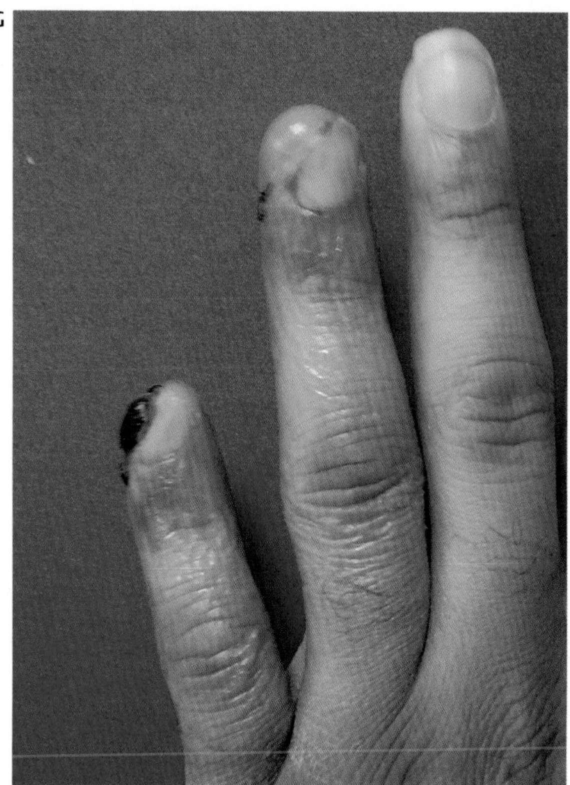

Figure 17–3 *(Continued)* **(G)** One month follow-up postrepair.

If the amputated tip fragment is unavailable, repair is dependent on the size of the defect and exposure of the underlying structures. Small defects of the tip (<1 cm) without exposed distal phalanx heal well by secondary intention. These injuries are dressed with xeroform gauze, and patients are counseled to perform dressing changes b.i.d. Large defects are closed with full thickness skin grafts from either the hypothenar eminence or the forearm. When the distal phalanx is exposed, the wound is thoroughly irrigated and local flaps can be employed for closure if the surrounding soft tissue is not significantly devitalized (**Fig. 17–4** and **Fig. 17–5**).

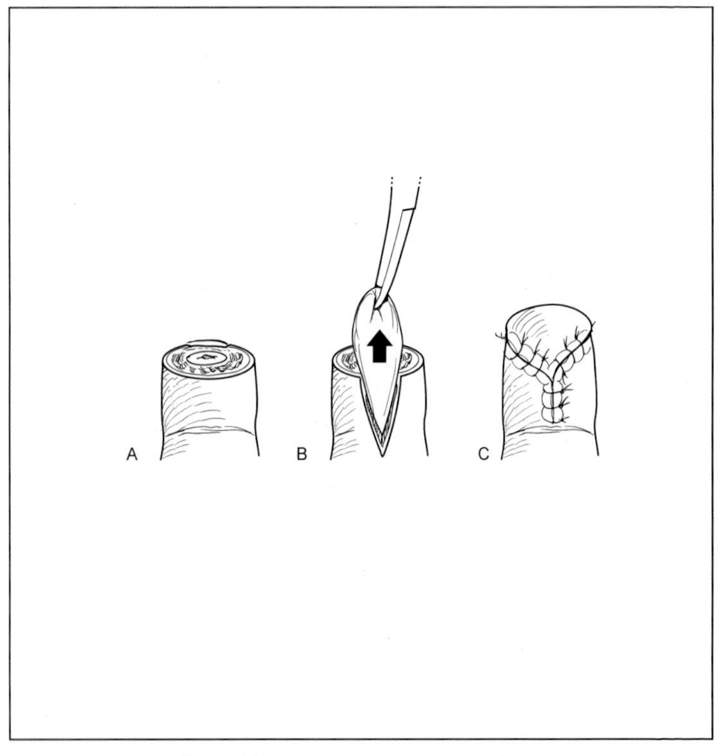

Figure 17–4 **(A–C)** Volar V-Y advancement coverage of transverse tip injury.

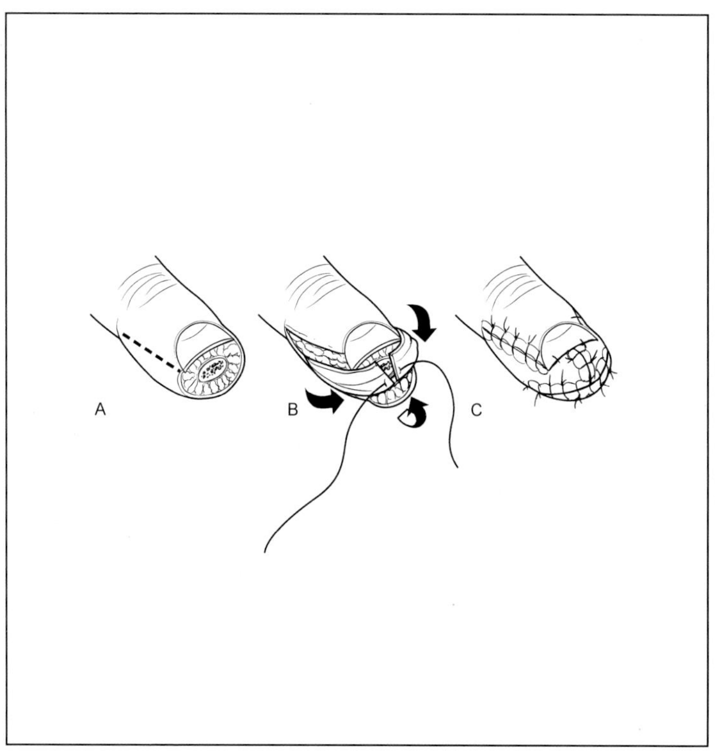

Figure 17–5 (A–C) Kutler lateral V-Y advancement flap coverage of tip defect.

Otherwise, the wound is dressed with xeroform gauze and local wound treatment is followed until declaration of the surrounding soft tissues. Short-term follow-up allows for assessment of the patient's wound for closure with local or regional flaps.

18

Upper Extremity Peripheral Nerve Injuries

Nerve injuries in the upper extremity occur as the result of a blast, a crushing or penetrating blow, or due to an injury caused by a sharp object. Management is predicated on establishing nerve continuity in an environment that will allow nerve growth and regeneration. Due to Wallerian degeneration that occurs at the time of injury, reinervation of the motor end-plates before 18 months will prevent muscular atrophy and subsequent deformity. Therefore, appropriate initial management of these injuries will confer successful results with minimal functional morbidity.

♦ Classification of Injury (Fig. 18–1)

First Degree: Neuropraxia

These injuries occur secondary to crushing, compressing, or stretching of the nerve. In these scenarios, the nerve architecture is not disrupted and there is nerve incontinuity. Conservative management including splinting of the involved extremity and physical therapy is appropriate. The nerve should recover in 3 months; otherwise, a second, third, or fourth degree injury should be suspected that would require operative intervention.

Second, Third, and Fourth Degree Injuries

Injuries that disrupt the internal architecture of the nerve may be isolated axonal derangement of nerve fascicles with subsequent

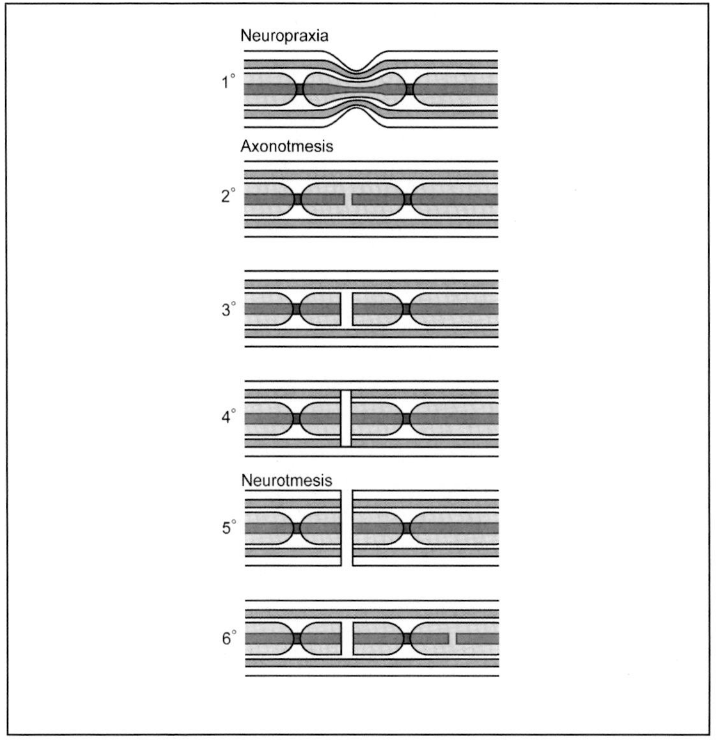

Figure 18–1 The Seddon-Sunderland-MacKinnon classification of nerve injury.

scar formation (axonotmesis/second degree). However, there may exist a scar conduction block at the fascicular level or across the entire nerve (third and fourth degree). An axonotmetic lesion will heal without surgical intervention by allowing nerve growth through the intact sheath at 1 mm per day or one inch per month. Injuries that heal with a scar block cause incomplete conduction across the nerve. These lesions may require internal neurolysis or excision and direct repair, depending on the conduction drop across the scar. Differentiation of the degrees of these lesions is determined by EMG and nerve conduction studies done at some time interval after the injury, if no nerve function returns.

Fifth and Sixth Degree Injuries

A complete disruption of the nerve is referred to as neurotmesis. Neurotmesis is repaired by direct coaptation or via nerve conduit grafts. The sixth degree injury is multiple lesions along the length of the nerve. Due to the potential longitudinal scar formation, these lesions require operative intervention.

♦ Management

The location of the injury is obvious in patients that present with peripheral nerve injuries. Commonly, the injury is open and associated with specific trauma to an extremity. Nevertheless, a thorough physical examination is warranted to determine the degree of function loss. The motor examination should include assessment of all involved muscle groups with documentation of their strength. Sensory examination includes the assessment of light touch, two-point discrimination, and vibratory stimulus.

The specific management of these injuries depends on the degree of injury and mechanism. Generally, closed injuries – neurapraxic or axonotmetic – are managed conservatively. Recovery of function is expected within 3 months. Open injuries are repaired primarily if the nerve and surrounding soft tissue does not have the potential for devitalization. Sharp lacerations of the nerve should be explored and repaired at the time of injury after the wound bed is decontaminated. Repair is delayed in blast, crush, and avulsion injuries. With these lesions the nerve is considered "stunned" with the potential for devitalization of nerve and tissues in the subacute period. Often these injuries are open. Therefore, the nerve should be explored and examined. If the nerve ends are in close proximity, the nerve is repaired. Otherwise, nerve ends are tagged for delayed repair in 4 to 6 weeks. Primary nerve grafting is not recommended in blast, crush, and avulsion injuries. In open injuries, nerve repair is performed after subsequent repair of bony and vascular damaged structures.

♦ Brachial Plexus Injuries

Injury to the brachial plexus is suspected in patients that present with high velocity wounds or direct penetration in the region of the cervical roots. These patients will present with gross sensation and weakness of the involved upper extremity. Care must be taken to rule out associated injury to the cervical spine and thoracic outlet vessels and shoulder girdle.

Evaluation

Physical examination is performed to determine the location of the lesion based on knowledge of the brachial plexus anatomy (**Fig. 18–2**). Examination includes assessment of sensory loss, motor function, and vascular integrity. In addition to the physical examination, radiographic evaluation of the cervical spine and involved upper extremity is performed. CT scans of the cervical region would reveal a cervical spine injury and assist in the evaluation for root avulsion.

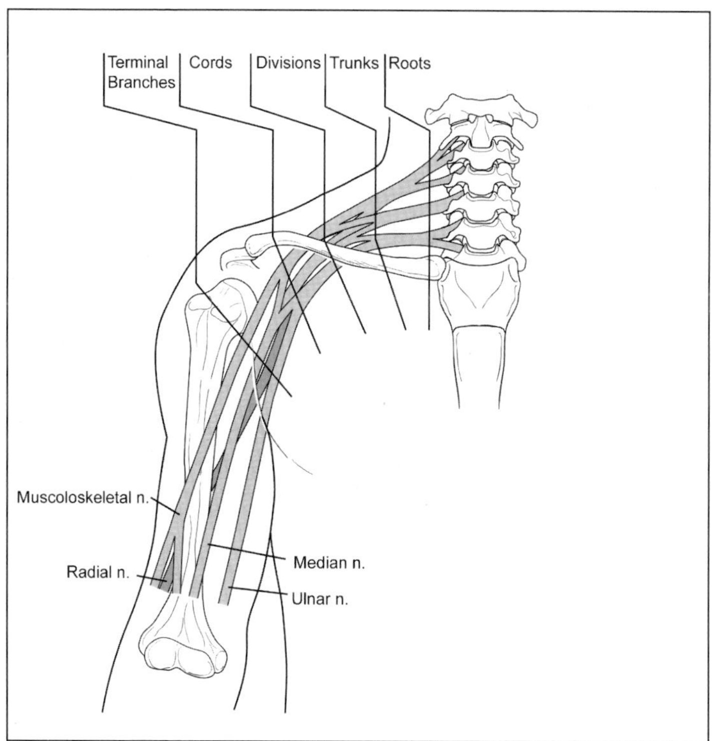

Figure 18–2 Anatomy of the brachial plexus.

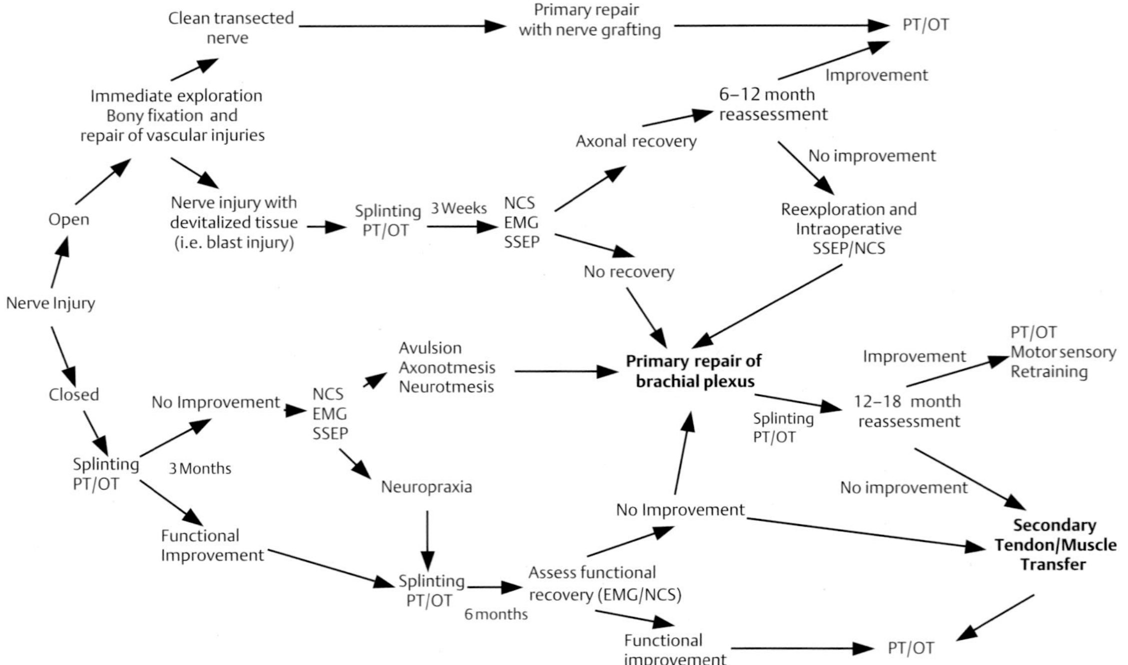

Figure 18–3 Algorithm for management of brachial plexus injuries. PT, physal therapy; OT, occupational therapy.

Management

Management of brachial plexus injuries is dependant on whether the lesion is an avulsion or a rupture outside of the spinal cord. Avulsion lesions will require delayed reconstruction after a thorough assessment of the functional anatomy of the plexus by EMG/NCS and SSEP studies. In the acute setting, these patients are treated conservatively with splinting and rehabilitation. The upper extremity is placed with the elbow in flexion and the hand and wrist in the safe position.

Lesions outside of the CNS (ruptures) are managed similar to isolated peripheral nerve injuries (**Fig. 18–3**).

19

Upper Extremity Compartment Syndrome

Blunt crushing trauma is the most common cause of upper extremity compartment syndrome. Although less common, compartment syndrome can also occur in the hand and fingers. When confronting upper extremity injuries, it is important to closely monitor the patients for tissue ischemia and to correctly diagnose those who develop a true compartment syndrome. Delay in surgical intervention leads to devastating consequences. Compartment syndrome of the upper extremity requires urgent care due to its immediate sequela of muscle ischemia and long-term sequela of Volkmann contracture.

Increased compartment content or decreased compartment size leads to increased compartment pressures that cause tissue ischemia. Pay special attention to compartment pressures in cases of crush injury, severe soft tissue damage, fractures, intravenous infiltration, injection injuries, arterial insufficiency, burns, snakebites, lying on limb, and *tight casts*.

♦ Diagnosis

The diagnosis of compartment syndrome is primarily a clinical one. The patient will have persistent pain that becomes worse with passive muscle stretching (a hallmark) or active flexion. The patient complains of diminished sensation, muscle weakness, and pain on palpation of the compartments. The presence of palpable pulses or Doppler ultrasound signals does not exclude increased intracompartmental pressures and compartment syndrome.

Cardinal Signs

- Persistent, progressive pain unrelieved with immobilization and elevation
- Pain with passive extension
  - Passive muscle stretch test
    - Forearm
      - Dorsal compartment: Finger, thumb, and ulnar wrist extensors – test with passive wrist flexion
      - Mobile wad: Extensor carpi radialis longus, extensor carpi radialis brevis, brachioradialis – test with passive wrist flexion
      - Volar compartment: Flexors of the fingers, thumb, and wrist – test by passive extension of the fingers, thumb, and wrist
    - Hand
      - Intrinsic compartments: Keep MP joints in full extension and PIP joints in flexion. Pain with passive abduction and adduction of the fingers is diagnostically significant
      - Thumb adductor compartment: Pull and abduct the thumb
- Diminished sensation
- Tense, tender forearm, or hand

Although a cool, pale, and pulseless extremity is often described in compartment syndrome, these are considered secondary signs and are often not present until late. Their absence should not delay surgery if cardinal signs are present.

Pressure Measurement

Use a Stryker needle (**Fig. 19–1**) or arterial line (**Fig. 19–2**) to measure compartment pressure. Forearm compartment pressures can be measured in the mobile wad and volar compartments with a Stryker needle:

< 25 mm Hg = normal – clinical observation, if worsens, repeat measurements

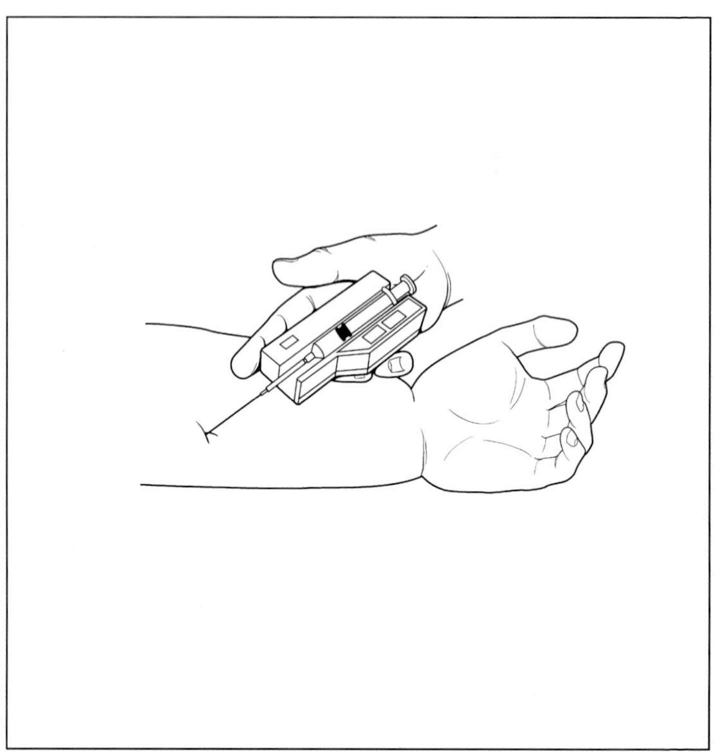

Figure 19–1 Stryker measurement of compartment pressure. Needle is placed in forearm compartment. Measure pressure of normal arm as control. Detailed instructions are on the back of the stryker needle device.

25 to 30 mm Hg = suspicious – observation with repeat measurements q2h

Normotensive patients with positive clinical findings and pressure >30 mm Hg for ≤8 hours Diagnostic for compartment syndrome

Altered mental status and pressure >30 mm Hg for ≤8 hours Highly suspicious for compartment syndrome

Hypotensive patients with compartment pressure <20 mm Hg below diastolic blood pressure for ≤8 hours Highly suspicious for compartment syndrome

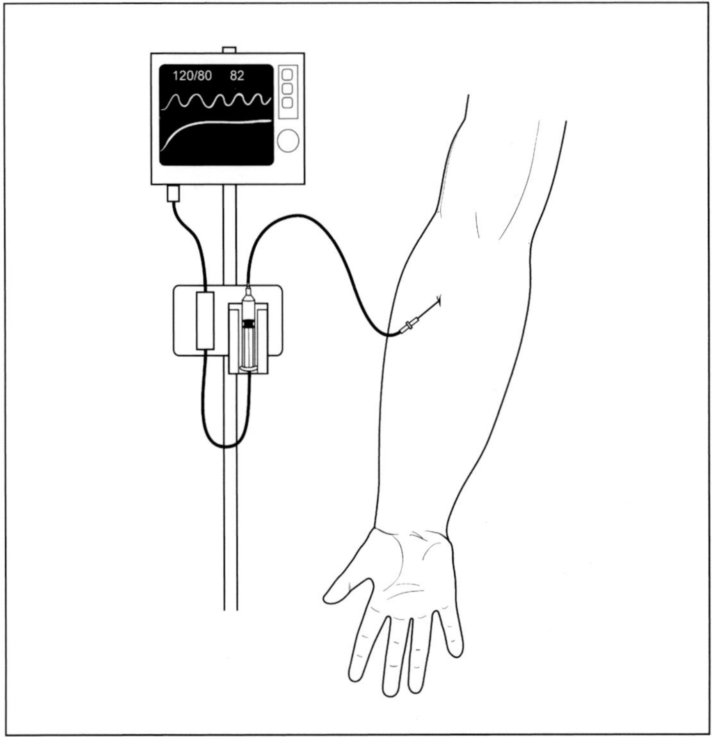

Figure 19–2 Measurement of compartment pressure with arterial line setup. Needle is placed into forearm compartment—not vein or artery. Zero the pressure at the level where needle is placed prior to entering the compartment.

♦ Fasciotomy

Perform a fasciotomy when the above symptoms are present or compartment pressures >30 mm Hg or if compartment pressures are within 20 mm Hg of diastolic pressures. Perform an immediate fasciotomy (1) if the time of onset of signs and symptoms is unknown, or (2) the patient is obtunded or unconscious. A prophylactic fasciotomy is performed if an arterial injury with ischemic time of 4 to 6 hours exists.

Hand compartment pressures are difficult to assess and often inaccurate. Rely on a clinical examination in making a diagnosis of compartment syndrome.

Muscle/Nerve Ischemia Time

After 8 hours, the effects are irreversible.

Management

Fasciotomy and release of the compartments is the only treatment for compartment syndrome. *Do not elevate* an extremity that has not been decompressed because the decreased perfusion causes an increase in ischemic damage. Elevation of the extremity after decompression is appropriate.

- *Number of Compartments* 4 in forearm and 10 in the hand
  - *Forearm* Volar superfical and deep, dorsal, and mobile wad
  - *Hand* Dorsal interossei × 4, volar interossei × 3, hypothenar, thenar, and adductor pollicis

Forearm Fasciotomy (Fig. 19–3)

Release median nerve, ulnar nerve and all three volar compartments. Check muscle bellies in superficial and deep volar compartment. Perform an epimysiotomy if necessary. Incision is started between the thenar and hypothenar eminence (similar to a carpal tunnel incision). At the wrist crease, the incision is carried transversely in the flexion crease directly to the Guyon canal and the ulnar nerve is released. Avoid transecting the palmar branch of the median nerve or straight incisions perpendicular to the wrist crease. Next, carry out the incision ~ 5 cm proximal to the wrist crease on the ulnar side of the forearm to create a flap for median nerve coverage. Next, curve the incision radially. The incision should reach its radial apex ~ one-half to two-thirds of the way up the forearm. The incision is then made in the ulnar direction to a point just radial to the medial epicondyle where it can be carried up to explore the brachial artery and avoids a straight incision across the antecubital fossa. The incision should be extended above the elbow where the lacertus fibrosus is released. If muscles appear necrotic, do not débride them because the extent of the injuries cannot be determined at the time of initial fasciotomy. Cover the median nerve with the small wrist skin flap. The mobile wade is released at the apex of the radial portion of the incision. After release of the superficial volar compartment the deep volar compartment must be released in an interval between the sublimus tendons and the flexor carpi radialis. This will prevent ischemic contraction of the muscles of the deep volar

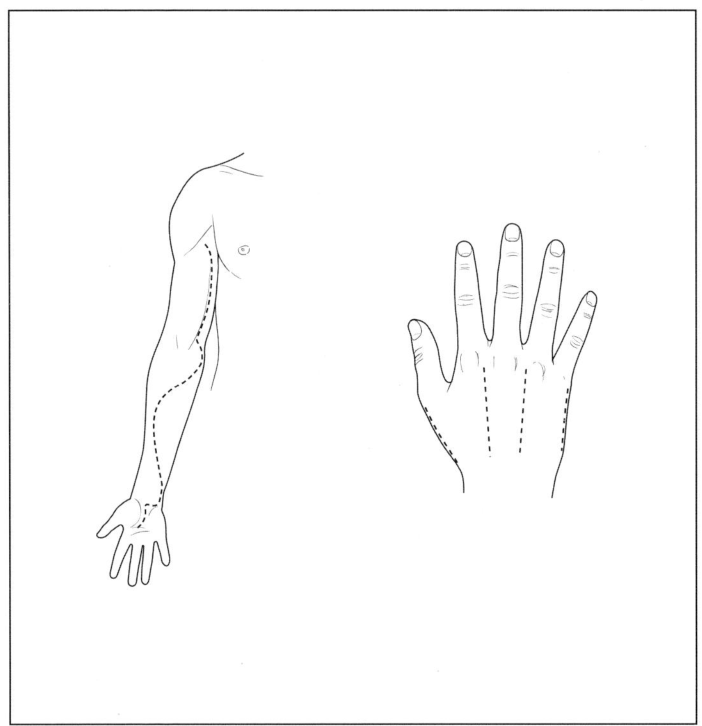

Figure 19–3 Rowland incision for forearm fasciotomy.

compartment. Release of the volar compartments significantly decreases the tension of the dorsal forearm. However, if significant tension in this area persists after complete release of all volar compartments, an incision is made along the midpoint of this area.

Hand Fascioting

Release the dorsal interossei, volar interossei, and adductor pollicis through incisions on the dorsum of the second and fourth metacarpals (**Fig. 19–3**). On either side of the metacarpal, release the interossei fascia and expose the muscles. Next, release the first volar interossei and the adductor pollicis, spread blunt tip scissors along the ulnar side of the second metacarpal. In similar fashion, release the second and third volar interosseous muscles by spreading along the radial sides of the fourth and fifth metacarpal.

Finally, release the thenar and hypothenar compartment using longitudinal incisions along the radial side of the first and the ulnar side of the fifth metacarpal, respectively.

Digits

In severe injuries or burns to the digits one performs a finger fasciotomy/escharotomy. Use a mid-axial incision along the nondominant side of the finger. The mid-axial portion of the finger is marked by first flexing the finger. Next, a line is drawn that interconnects the most dorsal aspect of the flexion creases to each other and to a point lateral to the nail plate. The nondominant side of the finger is usually the ulnar side of the index, long finger, and ring finger. For the thumb and little finger, release via an incision on the radial side of the digit. Then, release the flexor tendon by dissecting along the volar side of the flexor tendon sheath and releasing all vertical connections. Carry out the incision across the midline at the tip of the finger.

Perioperative Medical Management

Patients should be monitored for crush syndrome and the systemic sequela of massive myonecrosis. This is performed by analysis of serum potassium, creatinine kinase, and myoglobin. Additionally, the renal protective strategies are warranted. These include bladder catheter drainage and aggressive hydration to ensure a urine output between 0.5 to 1 cc/kg/hour. Additionally, assessment of the urine pH and myoglobin should be performed. In cases of significant myoglobinurea, the urine should be alkalized with acetazolamide (250 mg PO qAM or 5 mg/kg IV q24h) and mannitol (50 to 100 g of 5% solution IV over 2 hours, repeat dose to maintain urine output with a maximum of 200 g/day). Serial assessment of serum K^+, CK, and urine myoglobin are parameters to follow and dictate resolution of disease as well as termination of treatment.

Postoperative

Splint the wrist in extension, MCP joints at 90 degrees, thumb in abduction, and IP joints at 180 degrees. Elevate the extremity after decompression. No efforts should be made at skin closure; however, skin should be loosely closed over exposed nerves and arteries. Dress open areas with xeroform or Adaptec (Johnson & Johnson, Inc., New Brunswick, NJ) gauze followed with Kerlix (Kendall Company, Mansfield, MA) and a volar splint. Elevate extremity postoperatively. Maintain neurovascular checks in a monitored care unit to assess for adequate decompression. In severe cases, plan for a second-look operation in 24 to 48 hours to débride necrotic tissue.

Close wounds definitively by 10 days. If skin cannot be closed, then place split thickness skin grafts on the wound. Prior to closure, all necrotic tissue should be débrided. Alternatively, Silastic (Dow Corning, Midland, MI and Barry, UK) vessel loops can be used to slowly close the wound with tightening daily.

20

Postoperative Evaluation of Free Flap Reconstructions

In addition to the basic postoperative approach to any surgical patient, the patient with a free flap reconstruction requires specific attention to detect and prevent a potentially compromised flap. An important rule of thumb is to physically inspect a flap when there is any question of a change in status. Unless you are very experienced, any examination of a flap with a suspected change in status should be reported to the attending surgeon responsible for the flap.

♦ Assessment

Vital Signs

Heart rate monitoring is important for assessing pain control, intravascular volume status, and possible arrhythmias. Inadequate pain control is a frequent cause of tachycardia. Be sure to ask how comfortable the patient is and assess whether additional pain medication is needed. Watch for bradycardia, which can result from heart blocks or overuse of antihypertensive medications such as β-blockers and analgesics. Most free flap patients will spend the first night in the intensive care unit on telemetry, therefore attention should be paid to the tracing to rule out atrial fibrillation, flutter, or other arrhythmias. It is important to control these arrhythmias, not only for the safety of the patient, but to maintain the viability of the flap. Sudden fluctuations in blood pressure can lead to turbulent flow across the microvascular anastomosis or within the flap, which could lead to compromised perfusion of the flap.

Blood pressure should be monitored very closely in the postoperative period. Most free flap patients should have a MAP >90 and SBP >120. Of paramount importance is keeping the patient from becoming hypotensive. Hypotension can result in recipient artery spasms and venous stasis that can lead to thrombosis. Due to the prolonged surgery, insensible losses, and postoperative third spacing, free flap patients are usually intravascularly depleted and often require fluid supplementation in the acute postoperative period. Intravascular fluid status is most accurately represented by the patient's urine output. Free flap patients should produce at least 0.5 cc/kg/hour of urine (35 cc/hour for a 70-kg patient), but preferably 50 to 100 cc/hour. Patients suspected to be intravascularly depleted should receive LR or normal saline boluses. After the first 24 hours, D5 1/2NS at maintenance rate is used for the stable patient.

Patients should *never* receive diuretics to induce urine output unless there are clear signs of renal compromise in a well-hydrated patient. Likewise, pressors should *not* be used to treat hypotension. Pressors should be a last resort and only used when absolutely necessary (profound hypotension).

Hypertension (>180/100) can lead to bleeding in a fresh postoperative patient. Elevated blood pressure is most commonly a sign of inadequate pain control. Extremes in hypertension unresponsive to analgesics should be managed with low-dose antihypertensives (hydralazine 10 mg IV, or labetalol 10 to 20 mg IV PRN) to prevent rapid decreases in the MAP that can ultimately be detrimental to a flap.

Oxygenation should also be assessed with a pulse oximeter to keep the blood oxygen saturation >93%. In replants, the oximeter is a useful tool to monitor the replanted digit. When placed on the part, loss of the signal indicates arterial compromise, whereas progressively declining saturations are suggestive of venous congestion.

Hypothermia is avoided to prevent vasospasm. The patient's room should be kept above 70°F (21°C), with heating units used liberally if the room temperature cannot be adequately controlled.

Drain output should be closely monitored. Although drainage may be high in the immediate postoperative period due to expected oozing, a drop in output followed by a sustained increase may be indicative of venous thrombosis. Extensive drainge should prompt immediate evaluation of the flap.

Clinical Observation

Although refinement of microvascular techniques has brought failure rates down, it is the early recognition of flap compromise followed by immediate surgery that prevents total flap loss.

Always notify the attending surgeon of any potential flap compromise and keep the patient NPO should there be any need for operative exploration.

In assessing a flap, good clinical observation techniques are essential. To begin, always turn on all the lights in the patient's room and evaluate the flap's general appearance. Healthy flaps should be pink, warm, and soft with a capillary refill of ~2 seconds. Any other appearance is worrisome. **Figure 20–1** demonstrates a congested-free flap. Note that *pedicled* flaps are often congested postoperatively; this usually resolves with time (**Fig. 20–2**). A sign of arterial compromise is a pale flap that is cool, with poor tissue turgor. Check to see if the flap blanches and for capillary refill (2 seconds). If an inflow problem is suspected, an 18- or 20-gauge needle can be used to prick or scratch the flap to assess for bleeding. Check distally, proximally, but avoid the pedicle. Always approach the flap at

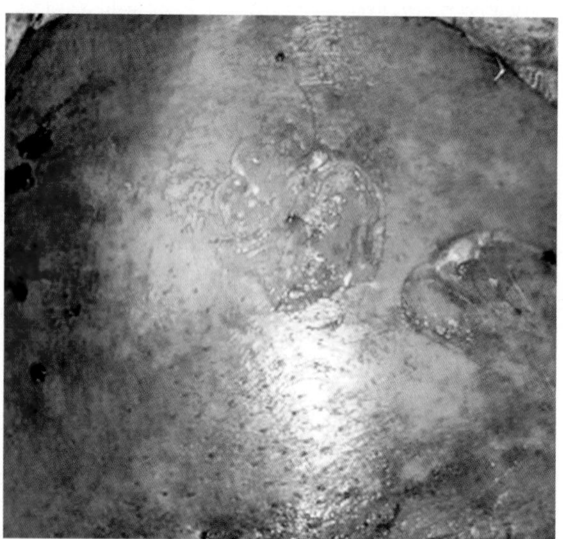

Fig. 20–1 A congested free flap.

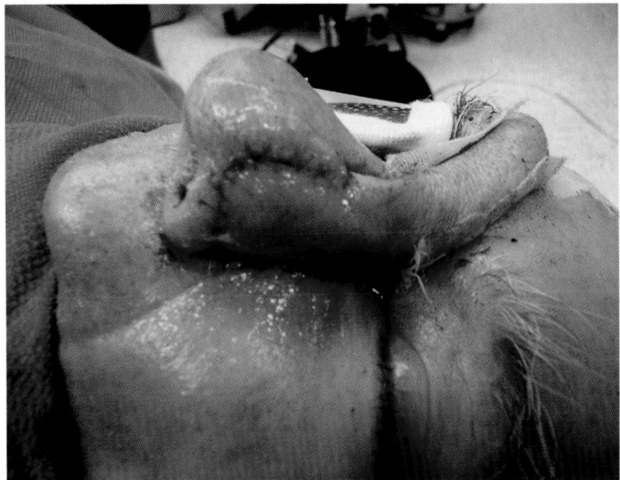

Fig. 20–2 A congested pedicled paramedian forehead flap.

a shallow angle to avoid deeper vascular structures. Signs of poor venous outflow are a tense flap with increased turgor pressure and purple color; the flap can be warm or cool. The flap will usually be oozing around the edges with venous blood and if the flap blanches, the capillary refill is usually brisk. A pinprick to the flap will also result in venous bleeding.

Doppler Signal

Doppler is used to measure the velocity and rate of blood flow through a vessel. Normal flow dynamics should possess three distinct audible phases. The first phase is heard during systole with the forward flow of blood distending the vessels. Early diastole represents the second phase where the elastic vessel rebounds and there is a momentary reversal of flow. The last phase is associated with late diastole and atrial contraction when there is once again a forward flow.

Therefore, any Doppler signal can be described as being monophasic, biphasic, or triphasic. Sounds should be clear and distinct. Triphasic signals are what one expects in a healthy flap. In the early postoperative period, the signal is often initially biphasic, representing the fact that the flap has been cold and ischemic for a period of time. As the flap warms and perfuses, the third phase will become audible. A monophasic or "jackhammer" type of sound is indicative of venous occlusion. Any change in the signal should prompt a very careful examination of the flap status.

Implantable Dopplers are usually used with buried free flaps, when there is no skin paddle to monitor externally. The Doppler cuff can be placed on the arterial or venous pedicle, but is more frequently placed on the vein. This is because venous compromise is more common and because an arterial signal can still be transmitted even in cases of complete thrombosis. A loss of signal is most frequently due to displacement of the cuff; however, a clinical exam should still be undertaken to assess the true status of the flap.

♦ Preventive and Salvage Techniques

Local factors possibly compromising the flap should always be considered initially.

- Loosen all constrictive dressings to avoid any unnecessary pressure or compression on the flap (remove sutures immediately if they appear to place undue tension on the flap). Sutures can be removed to help evacuate a hematoma, or to relieve postoperative edema and congestion affecting flap perfusion.
- Strip all drains to relieve clots that may prevent evacuation of a hematoma.
- Reposition the patient to correct any potential kinking or compression of the pedicle. This may sometimes lead to immediate flap viability and relief of compromised inflow or outflow.
- Elevate extremities when possible to assist in venous drainage from the limb and to reduce postoperative edema, both of which can lead to tamponade.

Anticoagulation

Leech therapy is usually used in digital replants or with mildly congested free flaps (**Fig. 20–3**). Leeches secrete the peptide hirudin in their saliva, which causes the flap to bleed. They can salvage a flap by relieving congestion. Leeches attach for ~30 minutes and actively suck blood from the flap. After they fall off, the bite wound continues

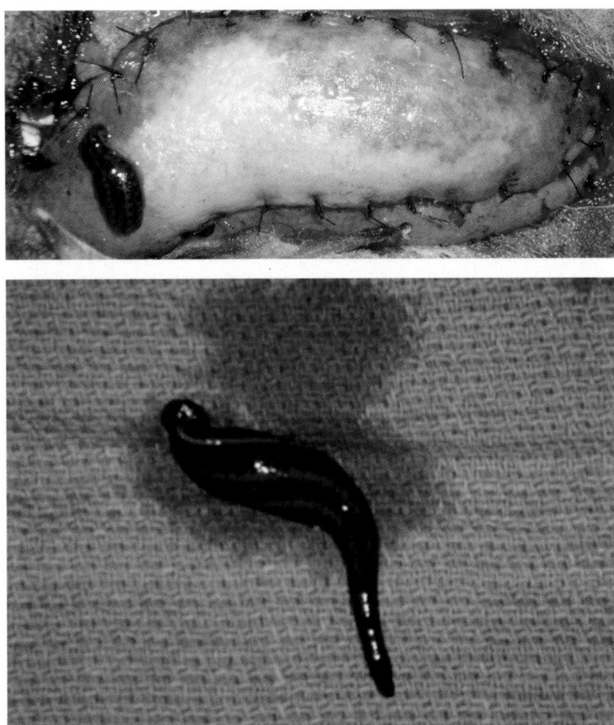

A

B

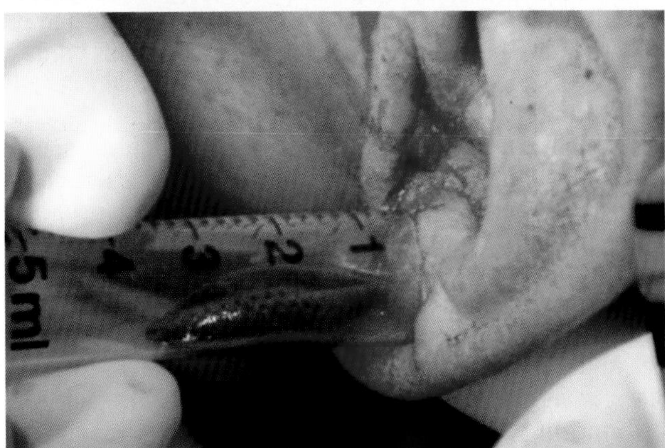

C

Fig. 20–3 **(A)** Leech therapy for a congested flap. **(B)** A medicinal leech (*Hirudo medicinalis*). **(C)** Use of a cut syringe for placement of the leech in the desired position.

to ooze due to the hirudin and accounts for most of the blood lost. When using leeches, the wound is more susceptible to *Aeromonas hydrophila* species and prophylactic antibiotics (Bactrim DS PO b.i.d. or Ciprofloxacin 500 mg PO/IV b.i.d.) should be utilized. If the leeches do not adhere, a 20-gauge needle can be used to initiate bleeding from the flap. This should facilitate leech feeding. After one feeding, leeches are usually sacrificed. Leeches can be obtained from the pharmacy, other local hospitals, or can be emergency delivered from Leeches USA Ltd. (telephone 800-645-3569). Although leeches may relieve mild congestion temporarily "a free flap that is congested should return to the OR for evaluation of the venous anastomosis.

Heparin is usually not used postoperatively, but can be indicated for some replants and anastomotic revisions. Full heparinization in the immediate postoperative period is associated with a fairly high rate of significant bleeding. In compromised flaps, a heparin bolus of 3000 to 5000 units can be helpful in preventing propagation of clot while a patient with a compromised flap is being prepared for the operating room.

Depending on surgeon preference, 10% dextran can be routinely used postoperatively. It not only acts as a volume expander, but also has antiplatelet properties. A 5-cc test dose is usually given and then empiric therapy is started at 25 cc/hour/day for 3 to 5 days or 40 cc/hour × 12 hours for 3 to 5 days. Side effects include congestive heart failure, volume overload, renal toxicity, and allergic reactions.

ASA is usually given postoperatively (325 mg q.d. for 2 weeks).

The use of thrombolytics has been effective in laboratory protocols; however, their use in the clinical setting has been mixed and controversial. They have been described to be effective in flaps with venous compromise to lyse thrombus within the flap. Streptokinase (500,000 to 750,000 units) 2 to 4 mg of TPA is infused into the arterial pedicle once the vein has been cut to prevent systemic administration.

Salvage rates can approach 50 to 75% if diagnosed early. The evaluator must be astute when assessing the free flap and keep in mind all the potential causes of flap failure (thrombosis, intimal flap, back walled anastomosis, kinked pedicle, tight skin closure, edema, hematoma, external pressure, vasospasm, hypothermia, hypovolemia).

One should not wait until the flap is purplish-blue, cold, and has no Doppler signal. At that time, the flap is likely beyond salvage. Always consult with the attending surgeon or a surgeon of senior experience after a thorough examination of the flap and be prepared to return the patient to the operating room if necessary.

21

The Postoperative Aesthetic Patient

In a postoperative evaluation of the patient who has had cosmetic surgery, one must not only evaluate the patient for early signs of complications, but also be attentive to the patient's comfort level, questions, and desires. Always check the patient's vital signs. A high heart rate, low blood pressure, and decreased urine output can herald an impending complication. In addition, ignoring high blood pressure due to pain can result in a hematoma formation. Hematoma formation not only may lead to life-threatening anemia, but also will compromise skin flaps and may lead to functional morbidity. Ask the patient if he or she feels pain more on one side than the other. This can often indicate a hematoma or infection – dressings should be removed and the wound checked (always remove dressings of patients who have had an otoplasty and complain of asymmetric severe pain). Assessing the patient accurately and proposing a concise and appropriate plan to the primary surgeon should be done prior to any intervention.

♦ Abdominoplasty

Considerations

- Jackson-Pratt (J.P.) drain's output
  - If the J.P. drain output is high and bloody and does not turn serous, consider a hematoma
  - Beware of low drain output and an enlarging/painful mass. Consider a hematoma. The drain may be clotted.

- Keep patient in lawn-chair or flexed position
    - Put sign above the patient bed to alert caregives of the desired position
    - Unplug the bed controls
- Incentive spirometry
    - Reduces atelectasis
- Deep venous thrombosis (DVT) prophylaxis
    - Get patient out of bed (OOB) with walker ± physical therapy postoperative day (POD) #1
    - Start Lovenox (Aventis Pharmaceuticals, Parsippany, NJ) 40 mg SC q.d.
- Abdominal binder
- Umbilicus viability
    - Small arms of delayed wound healing will eventually heal through secondary intention
    - Keep the umbilicus clean

Hematoma

- Diagnosis
    - Asymmetric pain or asymmetric bulging of incision/abdomen
    - Increasing heart rate, decreasing BP, and decreasing urine output
    - Dropping hemogram
- Treatment
    - Strip drains and check serial hemoglobin and hematocrit (H/H) (q6h)
    - Bolus fluids NS 500 cc and increase fluid rate appropriately (beware of patients with cardiac history – overresuscitation could cause pulmonary edema and heart failure)
    - Hold all anticoagulants
    - Type cross and hold pRBCs in preparation of transfusion
    - Operating room exploration

Respiratory Distress

Pulmonary Embolus

- Diagnosis

  - ABGs (arterial blood gasses)
    - Look for hypoxemia, hypercapria, and respiratory alkalosis
    - High probability when low PaO_2 and dyspnea
    - Check for calf pain and swelling – if DVT is suspected, then request a duplex ultrasound
    - CT scan of the chest pulmonary embolism protocol
    - Elevated D-dimer
- Treatment
  - If you have a very high suspicion of pulmonary embolism then start heparin drip
  - Start patient on heparin or Lovenox
    - Heparin: Load with 80 units/kg bolus and then 18 units/kg/h infusion; check PTT q6h and keep PTT between 60 to 90
    - Lovenox: 1 mg/kg q12h SC

Pulmonary Edema

- Diagnosis
  - CXR
  - Listen to patient's chest
  - Check CVP if available; if above ~12, patient is volume overloaded
- Treatment
  - Start Lasix (Aventis Pharmaceuticals, Parsippany, NJ) 20 mg IV
  - Check urine output to keep intakes/outputs (I/Os) negative
  - Re-dose Lasix as needed
  - Monitor electrolytes

Overaggressive Plication

- This may lead to decreases in functional residual capacity
- This is more significant on patients with a history of asthma or COPD
- Treatment
  - First employ conservative management by changing the patient's position and by respiratory core to include incentive spirometry and branchiodilators
  - Exploration in the operating room

Dehiscence

Small area

- Reinforce with nondehisced areas with Steri-Strips (3M, St. Paul, MN)
- Local wound care with wet to dry dressing changes
- Future revision

Large Area

- Operating room débridement and closure

♦ Breast Augmentation

Hematoma

- Diagnosis
  - Unilateral pain, swelling, and occasional fever
- Treatment
  - Strip drains if present
  - Small hematomas – observe if the patient is asymptomatic
  - Large hematomas – evacuation in an operating room

Infection

- POD 5 to 10
- Assess patient for either superficial skin or implant infection
- Diagnosis
  - Leukocytosis
  - Warm erythema along wound
  - Rule out periprosthetic infection
- Order ultrasound/CT
  - Look for fluid collection or stranding/inflammation around implant
- Treatment
  - Superficial

- Cellulitis can be treated with antibiotics
  - Clindamycin 400 mg PO qid
    - Clindamycin 900 mg IV q8h or Vancomycin 1 g IV q12h + Cefepime 1 g IV q12h for severe infections: also consider antibiotic therapy with equal oral or ID bioavailability (e.g., linezolid)
  - Exposed implant
    - Minor contamination without infection
    - IV antibiotics
    - Local wound care – Betadine paint
    - Plan for explantation with device change
    - Capsulectomy and pocket débridement
    - ± Site change or flap coverage in reconstruction cases
  - Infected implant (below criteria is controversial)
    - Plan for explantation and removal of contaminated prosthesis
    - Capsulectomy and irrigation
    - Delay implant placement for 3 to 6 months
    - Start IV antibiotics

♦ Rhinoplasty

Airway Obstruction

- Nasal packing or intranasal splint aspiration
- Aspiration of blood causing laryngospasms

Visual Impairment

- Vasospasm from local vasoconstricting anesthetic
- Thromboembolism causing ophthalmic ischemia
- Treatment
  - Urgent ophthalmology consult

Hemorrhage

- Localize source
- Treatment

- Packing
  - Gauze
  - Surgicel (Johnson & Johnson, New Brunswick, NJ)
- Endoscopic cauterization
- If all else fails: Posterior nasal packing (see Chapter 6, Fig. 6–4b)

Septal Hematoma

- Treatment
  - Aspiration
  - Incision, drainage and packing
  - Antibiotic coverage to prevent septal abscess
  - Augmentin (GlaxoSmithKline, Mississauga, Ontario, Canada) 875 mg PO b.i.d.

Infection

Local

- Cellulites
- Abscess
- Treatment
  - Augmentin 875 mg PO b.i.d.

Toxic Shock from Nasal Packing

- Postoperative fever, vomiting, diarrhea, hypotension without obvious blood loss, and an erythematous sunburn-like rash
- The supertoxin, toxic shock syndrome toxin-1 (TSST-1), produced by the organism *Staphylococcus aureus*, causes this syndrome.
- Treatment
  - Removal of nasal packing and acquisition of nasal cultures
  - Appropriate β-lactamase-resistant antistaphylococcal IV antibiotics
    - Unasyn (Pfizer Pharmaceuticals, New York, NY) 3 g IV q6h
  - Aggressive hemodynamic resuscitation

Intracranial Infections

- Meningitis
- Subdural empyema
- Cerebral abscess
- Cavernous sinus thrombosis
  - Diagnose with CT and treat with broad spectrum antibiotics
- Acute and/or chronic sinusitis
  - Treat with Augmentin 875 mg PO b.i.d.

Edema

- Treatment
  - Head elevation
  - Cold compresses
  - Blood pressure control

♦ Blepharoplasty

Retrobulbar Hemorrhage

- Pain, proptosis, ophthalmoplegia, ± blindness (See Chapter 6, Fig. 6–6)
- Treatment
  - If patient has visual changes
    - At bedside, open sutures and lateral canthotomy STAT
    - Decadron (Merck & Co., Inc., Whitehouse Station, NJ) 10 mg IV
    - Plan immediate exploration in an operating room
  - If patient does not have visual changes
    - Plan immediate exploration in an operating room
    - Steroids controversial
  - Control hypertension
  - IV 20% mannitol (1 g/kg) and acetazolamide (500 mg IV initially, then 250 mg IV q6h) can be used to decrease the intraocular pressure
  - If access to the operating room is delayed, and patient starts to loose visual acuity, then lateral canthotomy and cantholysis may be performed at bedside (Fig. 6–6)

Corneal Abrasion

- Diagnosis
  - Pain, tearing, and sensation of foreign body in eye
  - Diagnose with slit-lamp by ophthalmologist
- Treatment
  - Rule out a foreign body
  - Maxitrol (Alcon Laboratories, Fort Worth, TX) eye drops
  - Lacrilube (Allergan, Inc., Irvine, CA)
  - Ophthalmic bacitracin ointment
  - Resolves in 24 hours
  - Pressure dressing with eye closed for 24 hours

Edema

- Treatment
  - Elevation of head
  - Swiss eye therapy (cold compress)

♦ Rhytidectomy

Hematoma

- Most common complication, usually resulting from high systolic blood pressure, aspirin, or nonsteroidal antiinflammatory drug (NSAID) intake, or nausea and vomiting
- Symptoms
  - Pain, agitation, hypertension, neck/facial swelling, buccal mucosa ecchymosis, and skin ecchymosis
  - Can lead to skin necrosis
- Treatment
  - Large hematomas
    - Require immediate surgical drainage in the OR to avoid flap necrosis
  - Small hematomas
    - Evacuate at bedside by expression or serial needle aspirations and pressure dressing
  - Control blood pressure

Nerve Injury

- Assess the patient's facial symmetry by asking him or her to raise eyebrows, smile, and pucker lips
- Most motor nerve paralysis in the acute postoperative patient is due to local anesthetic effect, excessive traction of the superficial musculo-aponeurotic system (SMAS), infection, or hematoma.
- The most common nerve injured is great auricular nerve – provides sensation to the inferior ear and ear lobule.
- Treatment
  - Nerve paralysis immediately postoperative should be treated with observation. Notify the surgeon of specific physical findings to help determine the origin/treatment of the facial nerve paralysis.

Skin Flap Necrosis

- May first present as cyanosis and may be reversible
- Assess for hematomas, seromas, or infection and treat appropriately
- Partial skin flap necrosis
  - Apply moist gauze or antibiotic ointment
  - Treat full-thickness injury with conservative débridement and healing by secondary intention
- If patient presents with skin ulcers around the mouth, this may indicate a herpes outbreak and the patient should be started on Valtrex (GlaxoSmithKline, Mississauga, Ontario, Canada) 500 mg b.i.d.

♦ Liposuction

Fluid Balances

- Large volume liposuction (>4 L) can have large fluid shifts.
  - Monitor urine output closely with Foley catheter
  - Calculate fluid balance in terms of total in and out during the procedure
    - Input = IVF + wetting solution
    - Output = aspirate + urine output

- Fluid replacement
  - Small volume < 2500 cc aspirate
  - Maintenance IVFs only
  - Larger volume >2500 cc aspirate
  - Fluid replacement guideline below
- General guideline for fluid replacement
  - Total IVF supplement (cc)
    - Perioperative IVFs + Postop IVFs + wetting solution = 2x aspirate (cc)
    - Postop fluid replacement = 2x aspirate − [Perioperative fluid + wetting solution]
    - Titrate to urine output
  - Aggressive hydration will cause a hypervolemic state and subsequent cardiopulmonary morbidity.

Blood Loss

- Blood loss is calculated based on the wetting technique (**Table 21–1**).

Hematomas/Seromas

- Treat with compression garments
- May add further padding with foam or bulky surgical dressings
  - Large fluid collections that cause excessive skin tension and ischemia requiring operative intervention
- Seromas may be aspirated at the bedside or under ultrasound guidance.

Table 21–1 Wetting Technique to Calculate Blood Loss

Technique	Infiltrate	EBL
Dry	None	20–40%
Wet	200–300 cc/area	8–20%
Superwet	1 cc infiltrate: 1 cc aspirate	1%
Tumescent	2–3 cc infiltrate: 1 cc aspirate	1%

Abbreviation: EBL, estimated blood loss.

Lidocaine toxicity

    - Recommended dose when used at 0.05% = 35 mg/kg in wetting solution
- Diagnosis
    - Circumoral numbness
    - Metallic taste
    - Tinnitus
    - Lightheadedness, dizziness
    - Impaired concentration
    - Visual disturbance
    - Headache
    - Sedation
    - Tremors
    - Seizures
    - Greater levels of toxicity may lead to coma, or cardiopulmonary arrest
- Treatment
    - Supportive care
    - Oxygen/hydration
    - Maintenance of airway
    - Benzodiazepines for seizure prophylaxis
        - Diazepam 5 to 10 mg or thiopental 50 to 100 mg

Hypoesthesias

- Common and transient – sensation returns to normal within 6 months

Respiratory Distress

- Fat emboli syndrome
    - Intravenous fat deposits that cause pulmonary compromise and may lead to acute respiratory disease syndrome
- Physical examination
    - Tachycardia
    - Tachypnea

- Dyspneic
- Hypoxic due to ventilation-perfusion abnormalities
- High-spiking fever
- Petechiae over the trunk
- Subconjunctival and oral hemorrhages
- Agitated delirium
- Stupor, seizures, or coma
- Retinal hemorrhages

- Diagnostic studies
  - ABG – hypoxemia, increased pulmonary shunt fraction
  - Thrombocytopenia
  - Anemia
  - Hypofibrinogenemia
  - Urinary fat stains - Fat globules in the urine
- Treatment
  - Supportive therapy
    - Monitored care environment
    - Continuous oxygen and pulse-oximetry
    - Hydration
    - DVT prophylaxis
    - Gastrointestinal stress prophylaxis
    - Steroids
      - Decadron 4 mg IV q8h
- Pulmonary embolism and pulmonary edema
  - See Abdominoplasty section

Index

Page numbers followed by *f* or *t* indicate material in figures or tables, respectively.

F

I

V